Developing Primary Care for Patients with Long-term Mental Illness

Your guide to improving services

Richard Byng and Helen Single

with Catherine Bury

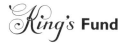

Published by
King's Fund Publishing
11–13 Cavendish Square
London W1M 0AN

© King's Fund 1999

First published 1999

ISBN 1 85717 271 X

A CIP catalogue record for this book is available from the British Library

Available from:

King's Fund Bookshop
11–13 Cavendish Square
London
W1M 0AN

Tel: 0207 307 2591
Fax: 0207 307 2801

Printed and bound in Great Britain

Cover photograph: Nancy Kedersha, Science Photo Library

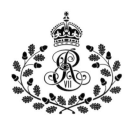

Contents

Table of Abbreviations   vi
Acknowledgements   vii

Finding your way through this book   1

1   Bringing the teams together   7
2   First joint working group: assessing need and
    developing visions for change   14
3   Considering options for change   26
4   Defining the changes in detail   49
5   Delivering and sustaining change   58
6   Improving communication   66
7   Facilitators' guide to change   74

Appendix 1 Good practice guidelines   91
Appendix 2 Prescribing and monitoring   95
Appendix 3 The Care Programme Approach demystified   98
Appendix 4 Needs assessment and audit with paper records   102
Appendix 5 Example of a shared care agreement   106

References   113

Table of Abbreviations

CMHTs	Community mental health teams
CMHW	Community mental health worker
CPA	Care Programme Approach
CPN	Community psychiatric nurse
JWG	Joint working group
LTMI	Long-term mental illness
PCG	Primary care group
PHCTs	Primary health care teams
SCA	Shared care agreement

Acknowledgements

I would like to thank the NHS executive primary-secondary interface R&D programme, which funded the research on which the book is based, and Lambeth, Southwark and Lewisham Health Authority, which funded the practices to be involved. Particular thanks go to Geraldine Strathdee, who has always provided enthusiasm for the work from its inception, and my wife Melanie, who has put up with my energy being diverted towards long-term mental illness.

Special thanks go to Catherine Bury, who worked with me as one of the facilitators on the project and was first author of Chapter 7, 'Facilitators' guide to change'.

Richard Byng

July 1999

Finding your way through this book

This book aims to provide primary health care teams (PHCTs) and community mental health care teams (CMHTs) with the tools to develop shared care. It provides a framework through which the teams can come together to develop services in order to improve the care of patients with long-term mental illness (LTMI). It enables the two teams to choose the most appropriate shared care depending on their interests, skills and resources. It is based on evidence, recommendations and the experience resulting from developing care in 14 practices in south-east London.

Chapter 1, 'Bringing the teams together' looks at finding a shared definition for long-term mental illness, provides a structure for holding a joint clinical meeting and outlines the purpose of a joint working group with responsibility for taking the two teams through the process of developing shared care.

Chapter 2, 'First joint working group: assessing need and developing visions for change' includes a look at the numbers of patients with long-term mental illness, an assessment of users' views and a description of the current roles and services of the two teams.

Chapter 3, 'Considering options for change' describes some of the models of shared care in further detail and looks at the advantages and practicalities of setting up case registers and databases. It also describes how this practice-based process fits in with the wider commissioning process.

Chapter 4, 'Defining the changes in detail' takes the joint working group (JWG) through the options available for the types of shared care, the roles of the various team members and possible service developments in primary care.

Chapter 5, 'Delivering and sustaining change' outlines how to set up a written shared care agreement between the two teams based on the decisions made by the joint working group, and then looks at how the plans can be put into action and progress monitored.

Chapter 6, 'Improving communication' departs from the focus on practice–community mental health team relations, recognising that important changes to the systems of communication need to occur at primary care group (PCG) or mental health trust level. The options for improvement are described.

Chapter 7, 'Facilitators' guide to change' gives a more theoretical view, describes the roles a facilitator might have in helping teams achieve their aims and then provides practical plans for the different stages of change.

The Appendices provide guidelines for care of patients with long-term mental illness and an explanation of the Care Programme Approach (CPA). A data collection sheet for audit and needs assessment and an example of a shared care agreement are supplied.

Introduction

People with long-term mental health problems suffer considerable disability and are at risk of relapse or deterioration. Primary and secondary care have traditionally been separated, leading to poor communication and lack of role definition. Furthermore, there has been no national programme aiming to improve service delivery for this group of patients. In recent times mental health has been an issue of increasing national importance, and there is recognition that care for those with LTMI can be improved further. The establishment of primary care groups and partnership boards provides a structure with the potential to influence care at a general practice and primary–secondary interface level. This book provides a framework for the decision making that is necessary to plan comprehensive care tailored to the needs of local patients, practices and community teams. It is designed for use by individual practices or groups of practices with similar views on mental health care, in recognition of the diversity within primary care. It explicitly aims to provide guidance for practices to set up the information systems necessary for improving quality of service and providing proactive care.

The book has been developed from research conducted with PHCTs and CMHTs in south-east London, from analysis of national research and recommendations and in consultation with other researchers in the field.

Objectives of this book

- to provide a framework for practices to develop long-term mental health services
- to improve communication across the primary–secondary interface
- to establish practice-based shared care registers
- to set up systems to identify and target patients not receiving adequate care
- to clarify the roles of the professionals for individual patients
- to promote training and staff development for mental health care
- to set up shared care agreements between the teams
- to produce a mechanism for monitoring and sustaining the above

Why and how to use this book

Each primary health care team and community mental health team will have different priorities and expectations. For some general practices mental health may not be seen as a great priority. In such cases the book will provide the tools for a rapid assessment of the situation, allowing clarification of roles and some minor service developments. For others, more substantial changes may be sought by both primary and secondary care. The book provides a framework to achieve these changes in a variety of ways:

- by carrying out a full assessment of the local situation, or needs assessment and considering models of care before deciding on any major changes
- teams may have strong ideas about how they wish to develop services – the assessment of the local situation could be brief but would be used to inform the planning of changes
- developing a reliable system for recording information and recalling patients would provide a secure foundation for practices to go on to provide some of the community mental health services currently

delivered by mental health trusts
- by using the principles outlined in the book to establish better joint working with social services and the voluntary sector; lessons can also be used to establish shared care in other areas
- practices could work together to develop shared care agreements
- PCGs could offer the framework as an option for practices to take up as part of their health improvement programme or practice development plans
- suggestions made in Chapter 6 could be used at a PCG level to improve communication
- the information developed from a functioning practice database could be used by PCGs to inform commissioning.

The book does not attempt to look at the hospital–community interface or radical new management structures for provision of primary and community mental health services.

The role of the facilitator

The role of the facilitator, if there is one, will depend on their skills and brief. Generally their aim will be to encourage participants to work efficiently and to focus on important decisions. They may be able to provide ongoing support and advice but will not be responsible for carrying out the detailed work. They will probably cajole a little in order to ensure the process runs to time. Chapter 7 provides a theoretical framework, plans for meetings and examples from experience.

Figure 1 Process for shared care development

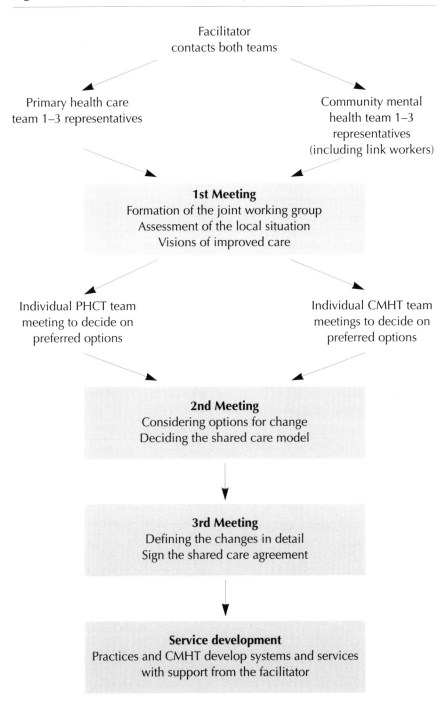

Facilitator
contacts both teams

Primary health care
team 1–3 representatives

Community mental
health team 1–3
representatives
(including link workers)

1st Meeting
Formation of the joint working group
Assessment of the local situation
Visions of improved care

Individual PHCT team
meeting to decide on
preferred options

Individual CMHT team
meetings to decide on
preferred options

2nd Meeting
Considering options for change
Deciding the shared care model

3rd Meeting
Defining the changes in detail
Sign the shared care agreement

Service development
Practices and CMHT develop systems and services
with support from the facilitator

Table 1 Examples of service development outcomes

Examples of contact details which could be made available to members of the PHCT and the CMHT:
- names, contact numbers and professional mix of CMHT and PHCT
- details of service provision for routine, urgent and emergency assessment
- practices' out-of-hours and crisis service provision
- bypass telephone and fax numbers

Clear definition of roles and responsibilities of primary and secondary services:
- clarification of the roles of the psychiatrist, attached/linked community mental health worker (CMHW), GP, practice nurse carers, voluntary sector and other professionals working for the CMHT
- who has responsibility for overall needs assessment, mental state monitoring, medication review, changes and repeat prescribing, depot administration
- PHCT involvement in the Care Programme Approach process

Communication:
- agreement on core information required by the PHCT in assessment, follow-up and discharge letters and by the CMHT in referral letters
- specification of a time period for receiving and sending letters, and the use of shared care records
- agreement on criteria for referral and discharge

Services to be developed or maintained:
- establishment of shared case register – criteria for inclusion and mechanism for updating
- recall system for review, depots and repeat medication given by practice, and joint team meetings
- guidelines for shared care

Staff training:
- agreement on training required, staff placements, and personal learning plans

---

Chapter 1

Bringing the teams together

Establishing a joint working group

Working out how services across two or more teams should be co-ordinated or developed requires detailed discussion, but not all key members can afford the time to be involved in the process. Establishing a small joint working group therefore allows for efficient sharing of information and ideas, and development and implementation of policy. The group will also serve as one reference point for both primary and secondary care staff.

Who should form the group?

Representatives from:

- the primary health care team (one to three members, probably including one GP)
- the associated community mental health team (one to three members)

and possibly:

- patients from the practice and/or representatives from a 'user group' (one to two members)
- a representative from social services, if they are not integrated into the CMHT

These representatives should have an interest in developing high quality services between the two teams. It is felt that a GP is likely to be needed as part of the group to ensure that decisions can be made on behalf of the practice. Practice nurses have skills in managing chronic diseases and are reliable in completing tasks. There may be a role for an administrative member of the PHCT (e.g. practice manager or experienced receptionist). Input from a psychiatrist at some level is necessary, but this may be through close liaison with JWG members.

Sometimes practice populations fall across two CMHTs' geographical boundaries. Clustering of practices to CMHTs is helping to improve communication between teams by ensuring each practice and all their patients are linked to one CMHT, overriding previous geographical boundaries. When clustering has not taken place or is not planned it may be useful for representatives of two community mental health teams to attend. Similarly if the functions of providing 'continuing care' and 'assessment and treatment' are not co-ordinated by one CMHT, it may be important that representatives of both functions attend.

There has been considerable discussion about whether users should join such a group. The progress may be slower but some practices and CMHTs may be keen to involve patients or users. It is important that the person chosen is able to cope with the demands of attending intensive meetings and can provide input at a policy and planning level rather than only offering anecdotes about services. MIND and other local groups have increasing experience of this type of advocacy and may well agree to provide representation.

In some areas, in line with Government policy, social services teams are integrated with trust community teams. If this is not the case, it may be useful for a representative to attend in order to make connections and to understand how the other teams are planning to work. It is also useful to clarify roles and working practices in the important areas of housing, benefits advice and community care assessments.

Breaking down the primary–secondary interface

A mental health trust in the north of England was concerned about increasing work load. It was struggling to meet the needs of those on the CPA register and felt overwhelmed by increasing numbers of patients with non-psychotic conditions referred by local practices. Its immediate reaction was to establish criteria for conditions that would be cared for by the trust.

Instead of taking this route, however, local managers and clinicians visited local practices to identify their priorities and problems. They then invited local GPs to help set up guidelines for care across the spectrum of mental health problems. This did establish that neurotic conditions should mainly be dealt with in primary care but also resulted in local training to help build the confidence of primary care professionals. Although this did not result in a reduction of referrals, the appropriateness improved and GPs felt confidant about having patients discharged back to their care. In addition, feedback on the quality and appropriateness of referrals provided by the trust was now willingly accepted by primary care.

Role of the joint working group

- overall responsibility for taking the process forward
- dissemination of the aims and objectives to all members of the teams
- consultation with all team members
- contact point for input from colleagues
- developing procedures to engage reluctant colleagues
- responsibility for drafting a shared care agreement between the teams
- monitoring and evaluation of the process

The group should be small enough to work efficiently and have a degree of executive power whilst also being able to consult widely. The work of the group would pause once the initial changes are agreed; they may wish to review the progress at three months and evaluate the process after one year, advising further developments as dictated by the changing environment.

Developing a shared understanding of mental illness

There are many definitions of severe or long-term mental illness, but there is no one universally agreed definition. In order to create a case register, the JWG will need to agree on a definition of long-term mental illness relevant to both primary and secondary care. All individuals meeting the agreed defining criteria should be included in the case register.

Our definition of long-term mental illness is based on the pragmatic concept of including patients with chronic mental illness often seen in secondary care, but who could reasonably be managed in primary care, together with those having more severe and enduring problems requiring a multidisciplinary specialist team. We have adopted an adaptation of the definition used by Kendrick *et al.* (*British Journal of General Practice,* 1994) and detailed in Table 2. Teams are welcome to refine the definition for their own purposes.

Table 2 Inclusion criteria for long-term mental illness

Patients having either one of the **psychoses**:

* including schizophrenia, paranoid psychosis, organic psychosis, manic-depressive psychosis and psychotic depression (excluding those with no medication and no episode/care needs for three years)

Or one of the **chronic non-psychotic** disorders:

* causing a substantial disability and having a duration of two years or more, e.g. recurrent or continuing major depression, severe anxiety and phobic disorders, obsessional neuroses, severe personality disorders and eating disorders.

    Duration: patient's disability must have been present for two years or more, including frequent recurrences or stable problems requiring ongoing medication or support).

    Disability may be defined as being unable to fulfil any one of the following:
    * being able to hold down a job
    * maintaining self-care and personal hygiene
    * performing necessary domestic chores
    * participating in recreational activities.

    The disability must be due to any one of four types of impairment of social behaviour:
    * withdrawal and inactivity
    * avoidance behaviour
    * bizarre or embarrassing behaviour
    * violence towards others or self.

NB patients over 75 years and under 16 years of age, and those having primarily drug and alcohol problems, learning difficulties and dementia are usually excluded, but practices may wish to include these groups in a wider register.

Holding a joint clinical team meeting

While it is necessary for a small group to do the bulk of the detailed work, the involvement and awareness of all team members is important. Discussion of clinical cases appeals to many that may not like other meetings. These meetings can complement the detailed work being done in the small JWG.

Receptionists intrigued

One practice agreed to hold a joint clinical meeting. The facilitator and community team members came prepared with notes of several shared patients and an introduction regarding mental illness for reception and administrative staff. This introduction had been specially prepared and was well received by these staff, who rarely had training on clinical issues. The second half of the meeting involved discussion of cases and the GPs were initially a little reluctant to reveal the names with non-clinical staff present as they had strong feelings about confidentiality. The cases were discussed in great depth with significant contributions from the receptionists, who had considerable insight into the circumstances of these patients. The GPs realised how valuable the session had been, not only to bring them closer to the community team but, more importantly, as an exercise to strengthen their own team. The receptionists all knew that they had access to similar information in their daily handling of notes but were amazed at being involved in such a discussion rather than overhearing it. Their training now also involves sitting in on GPs' and nurses' consultations.

Aims of a joint clinical team meeting:

- to discuss known cases
- to help raise awareness amongst staff
- to provide a good opportunity for the teams to introduce each other
- to begin the initial stages of creating a joint case register
- to promote joint working between the teams
- to use the meeting as an educational process
- to develop ideas for shared care to bring to the JWG

This approach has been tried with great success in Newcastle using the following guidelines:

- meetings were arranged to last for one hour, at a convenient time for both teams, perhaps replacing an existing meeting
- an independent facilitator was used with ground rules of confidentiality and no blame
- one to three cases of patients seen by both services were discussed
- the professional with most contact produced a brief A4 summary that was distributed before the meeting and briefly presented a case (one weeks' notice of the name of patients was given to the other team)
- other workers with contact added comments
- areas of positive collaboration and concern were highlighted
- action points regarding case and joint working were taken up.

Meetings of this type are different from Care Programme Approach meetings, which provide specific plans with the attendance of the patient. At this joint clinical team meeting or earlier, the aims of the JWG process could be available for distribution to all members of the PHCT and CMHT.

Planning for the joint working group meetings

A facilitator or nominated chairperson should contact the practice and CMHT to set up the series of JWG meetings, establish the membership and gather preliminary information about the current pattern of joint working. The clinical meeting may be before or after the first JWG. Any previous work on needs assessment, planning services or shared care could usefully be brought to the JWG, and this is outlined in the next Chapter.

Chapter 2

First joint working group: assessing need and developing visions for change

The process of working together to reach a shared care agreement may take about three one-and-a-half hour meetings, depending on the extent of changes anticipated and the initial degree of consensus. The meetings should, preferably, be facilitated by someone from outside of the two teams. Chapter 7 gives a guide to the facilitation that can also be used by a nominated chairperson if no facilitator can be found. Both teams will be asked to select members to attend the JWG and to agree mutually acceptable dates for meetings in advance. Members of the JWG should have access to this book at least one week before the first meeting. At this meeting each member will be allowed to express his or her hopes and concerns about the process.

Outcomes from the first joint working group meeting might include:

- a timeframe for the process
- agreed objectives and a vision for change
- discussion about the types of patients covered by any agreement (p.11)
- an understanding of patients' needs
- shared understanding about current service provision
- agreement about future meeting dates and work to be done before the next meeting.

Needs assessment for long-term mental illness in primary care

Why needs assessment?

Need has been defined as the potential for 'health gain'. As such, it focuses on and measures the 'unmet need' of patients with specific problems who are not receiving a treatment or some other intervention of known benefit. Originating from an epidemiological and evidence-based perspective, this definition is also valid from a more holistic and patient-orientated point of view. Thus, an assessment of need in general practice regarding patients with recurrent severe depression might reveal the number for whom regular reviews and prophylactic antidepressants are not provided. It might also show that those same patients wanted to be able to see a regular doctor and attend a practice-based users' group. Opinions of clinicians and patients are often qualitative descriptions, but are important and complimentary to quantitative data. This is an example of the 'corporate' model of needs assessment: by collecting the opinions of stakeholders a richly descriptive context is provided, ensuring that decisions to change and improve service provision are based on local priorities and interest, as well as an evidence-based epidemiological framework.

Needs assessment should not be seen as an end in itself; rather, like an audit, it is primarily a tool for improving appropriateness and quality of services, and is not just a box to be ticked in order to achieve clinical governance targets or ensure that a contract is fulfilled. The extent of a needs assessment may be determined by the willingness to change, the availability of resources and even the degree of uncertainty about the effectiveness of current provisions.

Table 3 Assessing need at a practice level: a summary of key points

Current services
- description of current provision
- overlapping services and roles
- missing services (based on evidence or recommendations)

Patients' priorities
- views on current system
- ideas for change

Health workers' views
- on current system
- ideas for change

How many patients?
- numbers on CPA register
- numbers with each diagnosis

Assessing unmet need
- numbers not receiving a review
- numbers not receiving an effective treatment

Information on current services

In order to plan or develop services, it is important to know about existing provision. While this may be obvious regarding your own team, when joint planning is being carried out it is important to understand the provision of both teams. The information collected also has immediate benefits in improving communication.

Which CMHTs does the practice refer patients to? Who are the CMHT?

Members of the PHCT will need to know certain facts about the local mental health services in order to interact effectively:

- sector names and boundaries
- any divisions within local services, e.g. for assessment and treatment

or continuing care

- who is in the CMHT, e.g. nurses, social workers, psychiatrists? What are their roles and contact numbers?
- the names and contact numbers of key clinical and management staff in relevant hospital wards
- a directory of secondary and tertiary service provision, e.g. information on treatments and specialist services directly available to primary care
- what the provisions are for routine, urgent and emergency assessment.

Information will also be needed as to the roles of staff relevant to the care of people with long-term mental health problems in primary care

- is there a linked psychiatrist? What is their role?
- is there a linked/attached community psychiatric nurse (CPN) or community mental health worker? What is their role?

Who are the PCHT?

Mental health services will need to know the following about their local general practices:

- who is in the PHCT, e.g. GPs, practice nurses, district nurses, practice managers, health visitors and receptionists?
- the names and interests of each GP and the extent of their psychiatric training
- the names of practice nurses and their experience of mental health
- the mental health professionals attached to each practice
- the current role of any attached counsellors or psychologists
- the referral and psychotropic prescribing patterns of each GP or the practice
- whether the practice has links to mental health group homes or hostels
- the practice's out-of-hours and crisis service provision
- bypass telephone and fax numbers, and email addresses.

Additional relevant information can be sought:

- what are the relevant local voluntary organisations?
- what are the contact details and roles of the local social services and housing departments?
- the addresses and contact numbers of group homes, hostels and landlady schemes.

Information relevant to each team can easily be collated in written form. An A4 card containing this information can be displayed in each primary care consulting room. CMHTs may choose to collect the information about each associated practice, to make it easily accessible to the whole team.

Current roles and responsibilities

It is worth spending a little time getting to know who is doing what in each team. The other team is often surprised about what is already happening and changes cannot be planned if the current status is not known.

Which professionals in each team, or elsewhere, are responsible for the following functions?

- overall needs assessment and recall
- medication review
- non-urgent changes to medication
- Lithium bloods and medication changes
- repeat prescribing
- depot administration and recall
- risk assessment
- mental state monitoring
- hospital discharge planning
- working with relatives
- providing benefits advice
- advising on sheltered or therapeutic work

The following questions may arise:

- is there any overlap of roles?
- do some patients miss out on care?
- is each responsibility clear for every patient?

Which of the following services are operational?

- practice register
- recall system for mental health review
- repeat medication linked to review
- depots given by the practice
- recall system for physical review (including health promotion)
- computer template/chronic disease card for mental health
- audit of care
- patient-held records
- local resource directory
- joint clinical meetings between teams
- computer prompts for evidence-based interventions

What do other members of the teams think about current services?

Ideas can be collected from the example memo below (Figure 2). This is an important exercise that is useful to further publicise the work being done on long-term mental illness and to assess the level of interest, as well as to obtain views on current services. It is strongly advised that members of the JWG consult widely with other team members about proposed changes before the next meeting (as outlined in the next Chapter).

Patients' priorities

A comprehensive assessment of patient's priorities can be gained from service users themselves. The insights gained can help shape services to become more efficient and user friendly. Finding out more about these priorities can be part of the initial needs assessment or a development that is carried out later. In the past they have focused on the following areas:

- access to services
- continuity of care
- social security provision
- meaningful daytime occupation
- support and social networks
- information on local services, diagnosis, treatment options and their likely risks.

Finding out about patients' views can demand a change in attitude as well as new skills.

The following ways of doing this are feasible:

- holding discussions or focus groups
- consultation with local user and advocacy groups
- informal conversations with service users during consultations.

Table 4 Running a focus group for users

Focus groups are a qualitative research technique which use group discussions to explore peoples' beliefs, views and experiences. They are particularly useful for groups of people who are not used to voicing an opinion, and/or who may have difficulty reading or writing. Teams are encouraged to consult MIND or SANE on help to engage users.

Size of group
The optimal group size is between 6 and 12 people. This enables group interaction to occur without the group becoming unwieldy. Participants should be seated informally in a circle to maximise interaction.

Holding the group
Group participants should include those with experience of the subject under investigation. Teams could thus use existing user groups or arrange for practice patients and mental health service users to attend. Attendance should of course be voluntary, with emphasis upon the confidentiality of the meeting. The group should ideally be held in a neutral environment, which is easy to travel to. The length of the discussion is usually between one-and-a-half and two hours, with a break for refreshments half way through the session.

Facilitation
Groups will need to be directed by an independent facilitator whose role is to maintain discussion in an unobtrusive manner. If teams have no access to an independent facilitator, a non-clinical member of practice staff with good interpersonal skills may be an option, e.g. senior receptionist or the practice manager. The facilitator will encourage discussion amongst participants by asking predetermined questions relevant to the topic under study. Facilitators must only direct the discussion and not become involved themselves. Doctors and nurses known to the group must avoid being drawn into a discussion about personal issues; their presence may be valued by some patients but may hinder open discussion.

Example questions:
- what qualities do you appreciate in doctors and nurses?
- what is the worst thing about coming to your GP or psychiatrist?
- what would make local services better?
- what kind of information would you like?
- would you find it useful to carry a card with a record of your medication and health needs to take to your different appointments?

> ## *Health promotion can make a difference*
>
> MW is a 52-year-old woman with a long history of paranoid schizophrenia. She is seen intermittently by a CPN or psychiatrist, normally in response to her daughter contacting the service when her compliance is poor.
>
> Two months ago she visited her GP, for foot pain. Uncharacteristically he was running on time and took the opportunity to check her blood pressure and smear status. Blood pressure was 220/112 and she was 18 months overdue for a smear. A longstanding vaginitis required treatment before an adequate smear could be taken and she attended regularly on time on several occasions; her blood pressure is now well controlled with calcium antagonists.
>
> This outcome resulted from chance opportunistic screening. It is now recommended that those with LTMI should have an annual physical health check, since morbidity is significantly higher in this group of patients. See Appendix 1 for a list of areas a practice nurse could look at in such a review.

Quantifying the problem

Before planning changes to services it is useful to gauge the size of the problem; a full epidemiological needs assessment requires significant work, going beyond the construction of a case register, detailing, for example the numbers with specific diagnoses and, more importantly, care needs such as the need for a multidisciplinary approach (CPA levels 2 and 3). This detailed work can be done before decisions are made but could also be one of the service developments resulting from meetings as a precursor for ongoing development. A detailed quantitative assessment of need using a computer system is only possible when you have decided what data you are going to collect, set up systems for data capture and run the system for a year! If you decide on a computer template to collect data for clinical use, the same data can readily be used for audit and needs assessment. Alternatively it is possible to collect data manually by going through each set of notes; clinical decisions can be made at the same time. Appendix 4 provides an example of a data collection form, which could be used.

In order to gain an initial estimate of the size of each patient group the following methods can be used:

- development of a *case register* to include those with long-term mental illness (See p.37). Local or national comparisons may be made
- gaining a *descriptive account* of how both teams see the priorities of particular groups and, e.g. ethnicity, homelessness, refugee status or local hostels
- *predicting numbers* of patients with major mental illness.

A GP with a list size of 2000 would expect on their list:

- 4–12 patients with schizophrenia
- 6–7 patients with affective psychosis (bipolar affective disorder and psychotic depression)

Figures for severe recurrent non-psychotic depression are not available. Practices in the inner city, near psychiatric hospitals and with an interest in mental illness will have higher morbidity, at the upper end of the range.

Quantifying the problem further

The following provides an example of numerical data that can inform decision making and planning for service improvements:

- number in each main diagnostic category, e.g. schizophrenia, post traumatic stress disorder, bipolar affective disorder, etc.*
- number in each CPA category*
- number on the supervision register
- number on Clozapine
- number homeless or living alone or in a hostel
- number from different ethnic groups

Additional information relating to interventions can be added to assess 'unmet need', as part of a more complex assessment:

- number with LTMI and no mental state assessment for six months
- number of women with LTMI aged 25–60 not up to date on their smear

---

* These can often be obtained relatively easily in first stage or preliminary needs assessment.

The last two demonstrate how audit and needs assessment are closely linked. The percentage of patients not receiving a mental state assessment is an 'unmet need'; the percentage of patients receiving the assessment can be compared with a standard set in an audit of care for LTMI. However this data is defined, its use is in improving the quality of care by demonstrating what is done well and what needs improving.

Table 5 Creating a case register

Individuals meeting the defining criteria may be located from the following sources:

Primary care sources
- request to each team member to list patients they can recall (see example memo)
- recorded diagnoses of schizophrenia, manic-depression, chronic/recurrent depression, other psychosis
- psychotropic drug prescriptions
- frequent consultations for emergencies/home visits
- depot injection administered
- hostel/group home/sheltered residence populations

Local mental health service sources
- case register of the long-term mentally ill from the CMHT
- Care Programme Approach register
- out-patient attendees
- CPN case loads
- depot clinic patients
- patients admitted under a section of the Mental Health Act
- crisis attendees, e.g. Accident & Emergency
- frequent in-patient admissions
- residents of hostels/group homes/sheltered housing

Figure 2 Developing a case register: example memo for other team members

Name ....

The practice/community mental health team is currently looking at its services for mental health care with the mental health trust/local practices. The aim is to improve the current services available. The first stage in this process is the construction of a patient case register of people with long-term mental health problems. A JWG will consider what changes in services can be achieved.

Patients will be included on the register if they fulfil the following:

Any severe mental illness (e.g. psychotic illness)
OR Non-psychotic illness with chronic problems and significant disability

Please write the names of all those on your case list which fulfil the above criteria in the space below. Focus particularly on patients who worry you because of their mental health. Think of patients who are significantly disabled by continuous anxiety, depression or personality problems, as they are more difficult to identify using computer searches:

....
....
....
....
....
....
....
....

In the following space, please write any ideas you have on the practice's priorities for mental health and on how to improve local services so that these may be considered in the JWG:

....
....
....
....
....

Please name a patient who you feel would be willing to share their views on developing our services:

....

Please return to .... **by** ....

Chapter 3

Considering options for change

Once the teams have met and shared their initial ideas for the development of services it is useful to consider the theoretical basis for improving the quality of care for long-term mental illness, the opportunities available in the current NHS, and the wider context of commissioning and service development. This will allow the JWG a more considered approach to planning change.

At this stage, the joint working group could consider:

- disseminating a needs assessment summary, ideas and dilemmas to all team members for consideration
- holding an individual team meeting to discuss major areas of changes with other team members. It is recommended that the options as laid out in Chapters 4 and 5 be considered. Preferred options can then be brought to the next JWG for negotiation with the other team.

Setting up a register

Gordon Place Group practice in the Wirral has established a disease register to develop services for people with chronic mental illness. Setting up of the register required additional resources to ensure the database was complete and accurate.

Patients with a diagnosis of schizophrenia, manic-depression, heroin addiction, dementia or depression that is still present after 12 months' treatment are included. Information about the level of disability and need for services is added later and recorded on an individual basis.

The register is used to ensure that additional care is offered to these patients. Patients on the register are offered regular, planned reviews of their mental state, social well-being, physical health and treatment, and are allocated a primary care team 'key worker' whose role is also to liaise, as needed, with other services.

Sources of information used to build the register include repeat prescribing data, data from the A & E department, long-term sick notes, CPN case loads, social services, all members of the primary care team including all nurses and receptionists, and hospital admission data.

The names of people with chronic depression are removed from the register after they have been free of symptoms for 12 months.

Pathways to improved quality of care

There are many competing theories, models and paradigms aiming to encapsulate the essential elements of high quality care. This model of service development has been developed from theories of quality improvement, expert recommendations, listening to grass roots voices in a series of focus groups and, most importantly, from putting the theories into practice and learning from experience. The book is based on a protocol for a research project, which took 14 practices through a service development process; this has been updated following that experience and in the light of changes in the NHS.

The available evidence base is scarce and rarely based on randomised controlled trials; most of the ideas and options espoused in this book are therefore based on opinion and experience rather than evidence. The objective of improving care for those with long-term mental illness in primary care often requires wholesale changes in attitude and practice. Furthermore, it is not possible simply to add quality control mechanisms, as existing systems often do not exist. This is at variance with two strategies for quality improvement programmes: to follow the evidence base and to build on existing practice. In the case of long-term mental illness it is unlikely that all the individual recommendations will be tested rigorously in the near future, so a model for service development was created drawing on expert recommendations and principles of good management rather than evidence. A joint working group of the Royal Colleges of Psychiatrists and GPs (1993) concluded that effective shared care can be achieved if some or all of the following measures are in place: close contact between GP and psychiatrist, integrated training, audit, locally agreed management protocols and well defined responsibility for control and monitoring of prescribing.

An additional guiding principle was that, since the components of good communication, practice guidelines, defining responsibilities, identifying practice and individual patient need and ensuring quality are often interdependent, an integrated package was required. A pragmatic needs assessment with an emphasis on local consensus and qualitative data starts the process, as systems for producing reliable epidemiology are unlikely to be in place. Meeting the other team with whom care will be shared and developing clearly defined responsibilities is at the core of the process. Audit and guidelines are not ignored but used judiciously. The aim was to produce a service development intervention which allowed flexibility at a local level while providing the support and ideas to avoid reinventing the wheel. Figure 3 attempts to encapsulate the essential features of the process.

Figure 3 Theoretical pathways towards improved health for patients with long-term mental illness

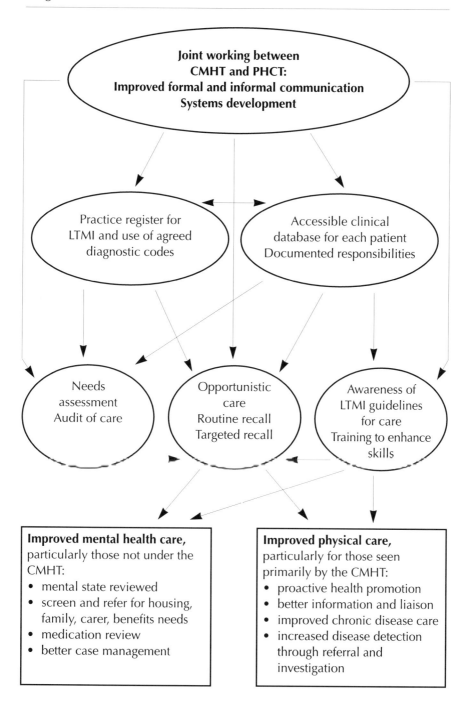

Models of shared care

Following the move of psychiatric care into the community, a number of models for shared care have been developed. Most rely on close contact and good communication between GPs and members of the CMHT. This is not an easy task to achieve, particularly in inner city areas with scarce resources and few incentives or contractual obligations as levers for change. It is also worth noting that there are one psychiatrist and two CPNs for every 15 GPs (approximately five practices) on a national level. The JWG may like to consider the following models, which are not mutually exclusive:

Separate primary mental health care teams. These are mental health care teams funded by primary care and based in the practice, usually with external psychiatrist support. They were occasionally set up under fund-holding and may see a revival with shared primary–secondary budgets in primary care groups. Their details are not considered further here but the work of establishing organised care within the practices and across the interface may be a useful precursor to this model.

Practice-based CPN. The CPN provides the main contact point with CMHT, providing interventions and advice, organising training, and acting as key worker to the majority of cases. This model has been criticised for allowing GPs to pressurise often-too-willing CPNs to spend increasing time (up to 80 per cent in one study) with non-psychotic patient groups, to the detriment of those with severe and enduring illnesses. Recent experience in inner city areas, however, has demonstrated how these CPNs have been able to prioritise psychoses in line with other CMHT members. With the current resources available it is likely that only groups of practices or very large practices will be allowed this model.

Linked liaison workers. Link workers are community mental health workers from the CMHT who are linked to practices and have limited responsibilities; they primarily act to give advice and as a communication channel for the practice. They are encouraged to attend meetings in the practice but do not preferentially take on practice cases. This is often the preferred option for trusts, particularly with the current recruitment and retention crisis. There is, however, little research to demonstrate the model's effectiveness, and it can easily develop into a sterile relationship as GPs and liaison workers have few cases in common. There is the potential for the link worker to become a barrier to, rather than a means of, communication. One way of overcoming this problem is for the link worker to have an explicit role to give advice about patients who are not under the responsibility of the trust. This may help break down barriers between the teams rather than building absolute thresholds for referral with the short-term aim of reducing work load.

Hybrid model. Community mental health workers from the CMHT provide advice to the linked practice but are increasingly taking on cases from the practice, as agreed by the team manager. This allows a meaningful relationship to build up through mutual cases while retaining a professional base for the link worker in the CMHT. It may be a particularly appropriate model if GPs are willing to take on the role of medical officer for less serious cases, but require the support from a specialised mental health professional. This will encourage a stronger GP–CMHW relationship, but requires team leaders to place cases preferentially (assuming skills are appropriate) with the link person rather than with the team member with the lightest load at that time. There should be a redistribution rather than a net increase in cases taken on by the team.

Shifted out-patient model. The psychiatrist conducts an out-patient clinic in the GP's surgery, mostly in the absence of the GP. This allows reduced stigma and can improve attendance, but has been criticised for failing to promote skill within the PHCT or to enhance real shared care. It is probably most appropriate in rural areas.

Consultation–liaison model. The psychiatrist attends a primary care meeting to discuss management of patients, after which the psychiatrist sees patients, often with the GP. This model is in some ways similar to the linked liaison and hybrid models, but with the psychiatrist as the link person. It has been deemed successful by both psychiatrists and GPs who have experienced it, and can be a good way of transferring skills to primary care. It is costly and could be adapted for use as a short-term initiative to enhance skills and communication as part of a wider strategy for shared care.

Traditional one-to-one model. Over time the teams get to know each other so well that they are able to choose the most appropriate member of the other team to talk to. With high levels of staff turn-over it often falls down, but at best it can lead to efficient continuity of care. The principle of encouraging one-to-one communication with the most appropriate team member can be included in the above models, particularly if information about team members and contact details are regularly updated and shared.

Within any model, decisions will be needed regarding:

- responsibilities for core tasks such as mental state monitoring, medication review, repeat prescribing and individuals' needs assessment (see Chapter 4 for details)
- which shared care relationships will be dominant or need developing, e.g. GP–community mental health worker, psychiatrist–GP, community mental health worker–practice nurse
- whether patient preference will be used to determine the main location of the professional/team for follow up
- the types of patient GPs want to provide care for.

Clustering of GPs or geographical sectors for CMHTs

The development of CMHTs has changed the face of out-patient psychiatry. Initially geographically sectorised, there is now a trend, established in Scotland, for CMHTs to work with clusters of GPs wherever their patients live. This has enhanced relationships between primary care and community mental health professionals. It is likely to continue with the development of relationships between PCGs and CMHTs. The hand over of patients as a result of any changes in responsibility needs to be carefully managed on a case-by-case basis.

Case registers

Case registers can be used to provide more preventative care for people with long-term mental health problems. They also lead to more effective collaboration between primary and secondary services and improved continuity of shared care. The services and systems the practice and CMHT decide to operate determine the function of the case register. The decisions about roles and responsibilities and service developments detailed in Chapter 4 will therefore influence the aims of the register and how it is constructed. The register may act in the following ways:

- as an accessible database for clinical decision making
- as a tool to organise mental health reviews for those not seen by CMHT
- to organise annual physical health checks
- to notify staff of missed medication/depot collection
- to enable people to be included in the Care Programme Approach and remind staff of forthcoming reviews
- to facilitate monitoring of repeat psychotropic medication prescriptions
- to facilitate audit of care input
- to inform GPs of the number and the needs of patients and to highlight those not receiving adequate service input (i.e. acting as a needs assessment)
- to allow the monitoring of resources
- to collect socio-demographic and service usage data.

Figure 4 shows how data flow and can be used in primary care.

Proactive mental health reviews

EG is a 40-year-old single unemployed man with long-standing depression. He had been seen regularly by psychiatrists during the 1980s, and was relatively well when discharged. He had been seen for certificates and medication, as well as minor illnesses for eight years when his GP decided to do a mental health assessment. EG was found to have moderate depressive symptoms, a mild paranoia of not quite delusional intensity and increasing financial problems.

A referral back to the psychiatrist with a specific request for advice on treatment, and a referral to the Citizens Advice Bureaux was made. EG is now on a different antidepressant with a low dose of Fluanxol and feels better than he has for years. The CAB have given him confidence to manage his finances and he is getting out more to meet acquaintances.

Figure 4 Information flows and the uses of data in primary care

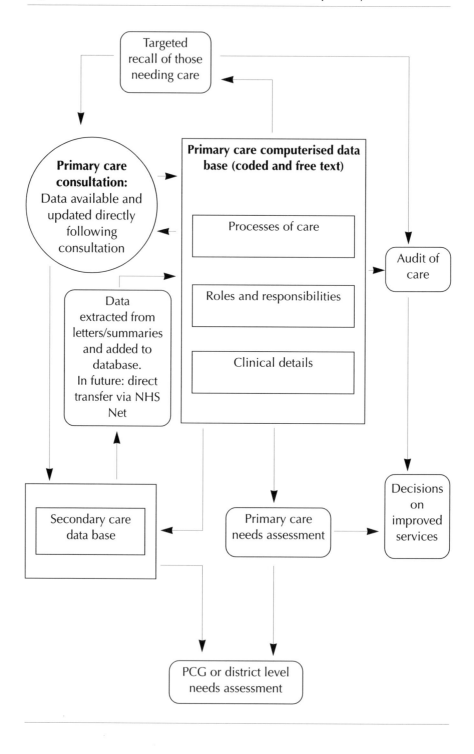

Table 6 Information that could be recorded on the case register/database

Case registers and associated databases may be paper or computer-based and over time the following information may be added. Page 44 gives a guide to planning data entry for each item, depending on your needs.

Socio-demographic data
Name, age, sex
Address, telephone no.
Marital status: *married, single, separated, widowed, divorced*
Ethnicity: e.g. *Asian, black, white, other*
Housing type: *council, housing association, rented, owned, hostel, no fixed abode*
Home situation: *lives alone – with help, lives alone – no help, lives with partner, lives with family, single parent*
Number of children/dependants
Next of kin/address/telephone no.
Neighbour/main carer/address/telephone no.

Accumulated clinical data
Diagnosis
Date of diagnosis
Previous Mental Health Act section: *types and dates*
History of deliberate self-harm
History of harm to others
Substance misuse: *alcohol, opiates, benzodiazepines, other*
Specific indicators of relapse
Specific crisis response
CPA level: *1, 2, 3, not specified/date*
Supervision register: *Y/N; date*
Section 117: *date*

Service contact
Normal GP
CMHT: *name*
Psychiatrist
CPN
Care co-ordinator/key worker
Social worker
Housing worker
Other involved agency 1: *telephone no.*
Involved agency 2: *telephone no.*
Involved agency 3: *telephone no.*

Sharing of care
Main care: *CMHT, GP, GP–CMHW, Psychiatrist–GP, CMHT–GP (first partner responsible for overall needs assessment, recall, if required, mental state monitoring, risk assessment, medication review and non-urgent changes to medication)*

Other responsibilities, which may differ from the above:
- Lithium bloods
- Lithium medication changes
- repeat prescribing
- depot administration and recall

Recall policy
Frequency of reviews
Date of next review

Data input required on ongoing basis when patient is seen in primary care or from letter of secondary care contacts (minimum annual)
Mental state reviewed: *completed/not completed*
Current mental state
Current risk of deliberate self-harm
Current risk of harm to others
Risk of self-neglect
Medication reviewed
Compliance
Date depot given
Lithium levels checked
Accommodation needs assessed *(can be linked to housing type and home situation)*
Benefits assessment: *date and outcome*
Physical care review: *completed/not completed*
Next physical review due

(Adapted, with the author's permission, from Strathdee *et al. A General Practitioner's Guide to Managing Long-term Mental Health Disorders.* The Sainsbury Centre for Mental Health, 1996.)

Constructing and maintaining a register using a practice-based computer system

Your objectives need to be clear:

- to have an up to date register of patients with long-term mental health problems
- link to a computer template/chronic disease record for easy access to clinical data
- for audit and needs assessment
- link to a recall system

If you use the computer to input major diagnoses and would like to recall patients with mental health problems, it may be worthwhile constructing and maintaining a system. Once familiar with doing searches it is not a difficult task. This description of constructing a register is based on the definition of LTMI outlined in this book. You may wish to use different criteria.

Stage I: separate searches to develop a register

Obtain names from as many different sources as possible: practice and CMHT, paper and computer-based and from memory (see also 'Creating a case register', Table 5 on page 24). The following lists might emerge:

1 Patients known to team members (using the memo is particularly useful for those with recurrent depression or severe anxiety where computer searches are inefficient)
2 Patients known to secondary services, e.g. on CPA or other case load register available from the CMHT
3 Patients likely to have LTMI, according to your computer database. The accuracy will depend on how much you use the computer. If it is used either for major diagnoses or for repeat medication then you will find most patients this way. Try to work out which Read codes you use on the computer and use these on the search. Some systems allow you to identify which codes are commonly used.

Different computer systems have different methods for searches. Some allow multiple diagnoses or medications to go on the same search, others require individual searches to be done for each diagnosis. Some practices will be very familiar with searches, while others may need assistance from the appropriate help desk.

Some systems allow searches for a Read code and give the option of including all or some of the codes in the level below (examples are given here for ICD Read version 5; see Figure 5 for other equivalent codes). For example, to search for 'Schizophrenia'-E10 is easy as all codes under E1 are types of schizophrenia and can be included. Affective disorders are more difficult, however, since, for example, 'depression single episode'-E112 comes under 'affective psychosis'-E11 in the Read hierarchy, which, like 'schizophrenia' comes under 'non-organic psychosis'-E1. If 'depression single episode'-E11 is used in the practice for single episodes of depression (non-severe) it needs excluding from the search. Other systems will only search on specific codes, one at a time. This may take a little longer but can be delegated to a skilled receptionist or computer manager.

Recommended strategy for computer search

Subjects to search on include:

1   Past drugs, e.g. all anti-psychotic medication prescribed in the last two years plus Lithium (and possibly Carbamazepine), Procyclidine and Orphenadrine. *Be careful to exclude Prochlorperazine 5 mg or you get a list of everyone who has had Stemetil!* If searching by individual drug, then those listed in Table 7 are the most commonly prescribed. You may know of other practice or local psychiatrists' preferences
2   Current drugs, as above
3   Non-organic psychosis, i.e. for Read version 5, E1 and below (except E112), Eu2 and Eu3I. If the system only allows single code searches, then use the most commonly used codes.

Table 7 Database search for drugs commonly used in the treatment of psychoses

---

Oral preparations
- Chlorpromazine (commonly prescribed as Largactil)
- Halperidol (commonly prescribed as Haldol)
- Trifluoperazine (commonly prescribed as Stelazine)
- Risperidone
- Sulpiride
- Thioridazine
- Olanzapine

Medication used for bipolar and unipolar affective disorders
- Lithium Hydrochloride
- Carbamazepine (note: exclude epilepsy and trigeminal neuragia)

Anti-cholinergics
- Procyclidine (commonly prescribed as Kemadrin)
- Orphenadine (commonly prescribed as Disipal)

Other drugs worth searching for
- Loxapine, Pimozide, Droperidol, Pericyazine, Zuclopenthixol

Depot medication
- Fluphenazine Decanoate (commonly prescribed as Modecate)
- Flupenthixol Decanoate (commonly prescribed as Depixol)

Figure 5 Simplified hierarchy for mental health Read codes (Version 5)

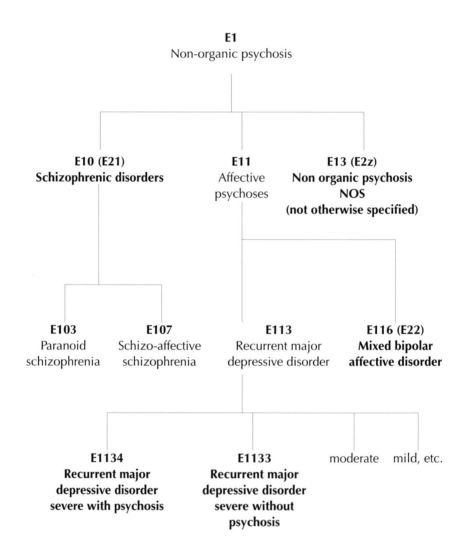

(Bold codes are those recommended for use on register. Codes in brackets are Read version 4. No code for recurrent depression is available in Read version 4, so we recommend creating your own.)

Stage II: choosing a limited set of diagnoses and combining to one database

We suggest using a limited number of diagnoses to define the register. Most practice systems use Read codes 4 and 5. These have obvious shortfalls but the alternative is to create a new system, which is too time consuming for an individual practice. See Figure 5, which shows a simplified version of the Read 5 hierarchy for mental illness and the recommended codes for the register. By choosing a relatively high level Read code and allocating a diagnosis to each patient it is easy to create a self-updating register – as long as a diagnosis is allocated! If you feel uncomfortable with Read codes or diagnostic labelling you could create a code to allocate to all patients, e.g. 'long-term mental health problem'. Patients may have more than one diagnosis, and hence code; as long as one of the codes is part of your list of codes which makes up the register it does not matter.

Those who are difficult to label can be given a non-specific high level Read code, such as 'psychosis NOS (not otherwise specified)'-E13. We have chosen E0, 1, 2, 3, Read codes, but you could choose the Eu codes, e.g. (X) bipolar affective disorder-Eu31, which are ICD10 equivalent.

Discussion between practices in south Lewisham has generated groupings of patients who may be included in a register for severe and long-term mental illness as shown in Table 8. Consistent records in primary care would allow for PCG level needs assessment.

In most computer systems any patient with a specific code, e.g. paranoid schizophrenia-E103 can be found on a search for higher level code, e.g. schizophrenic disorders-E10, so it is possible to create a register with some clinicians using detailed (lower level) codes and others using less specific diagnoses, as long as the same branch is used. For example, (X) schizophrenia-Eu20 would not be picked up on a search for schizophrenic disorders-E10. You must either agree a more complex search strategy or for clinicians to code consistently, e.g. a practice agreement not to use (X) type diagnoses for actively psychotic or ill patients. The templates or databases may also need to be actively linked to the chosen codes, providing a further incentive to limiting the numbers.

Once you have agreed codes for patients with long-term mental illness the search lists need to be examined and each patient given a diagnosis from the accepted list. One person can do this from the notes (a data input person with reference to a GP may be appropriate). At this point it is worth considering collating other relevant information from the notes being examined onto a computer template/database or chronic disease card, so that the notes do not need to be examined twice.

By searching on the high level codes agreed by the practice, e.g. E10, E116, E1134, E1133, E13, and codes for chronic severe anxiety/OCD/PTSD, a list of LTMI is formed.

Table 8 Groupings of patients with long-term mental illness

Schizophrenia
- Read 5 – schizophrenic disorders-E10 or
- Read 4 – schizophrenic disorders-E21 or
- ICD10 (Read 5) – schizophrenia and others-Eu2

(This includes lower codes such as paranoid schizophrenia and schizoaffective schizophrenia.)

Bipolar affective disorders
- Read 5 – mixed bipolar affective disorder-E116
- Read 4 – manic-depressive disorder-E22
- ICD10 (Read 5) – bipolar affective disorder-Eu31

Psychosis NOS (not otherwise specified)
- Read 5 – psychosis NOS-E13
- Read 4 – psychosis NOS-E2z
- ICD10 (Read 5) – psychosis NOS-Eu2z

(This includes those with psychosis and no defined diagnosis.)

Psychotic depression
- Read 5 – recurrent major depressive disorder, severe, with psychosis-E1134
- Read 5 – single episode psychotic depressive disorder-E11

Severe depression (non-psychotic)
- Read 5 – recurrent major depressive disorder, severe, without psychosis-E1133
(Severe recurrent depression and severe single episode causing substantial disability over a period of one year or more.)

Severe neuroses
Chronic severe anxiety, post traumatic stress disorder (PTSD), severe eating disorders and obsessive compulsive disorder (OCD) can all produce long-term disability. This grouping has not been discussed fully.

An alternative grouping would include schizophrenia and unspecified psychosis under 'chronic psychosis' and psychotic depression and bipolar disorder under 'affective psychoses'.

Stage III: updating the register

1 Use the above codes for clinical day-to-day use and when coding diagnoses from out-patient and discharge letters

2 A quarterly search on drugs and miscellaneous mental health codes as an initial search, but excluding codes being used for the register, will give you a list of names to consider adding to the register. This option is available on Meditel and Emis systems

3 Patients may need to be removed from the register if their problem no longer merits active management. One solution is to recode them as a diagnosis not included on the register. For example, the (X) codes could be used for denoting past histories: the computer record will still show an accurate diagnosis but the register will not include those with a past history but no current care needs.

Planning data entry for each patient's clinical database

The database for each patient needs to provide the functions of audit, needs assessment and, most importantly, an accessible source of clinical data. The data entry system or template therefore needs to be created with these in mind. Categorising and coding different aspects of health and care is important. Each of the domains in Table 6 above needs to be considered with respect to these three main functions. For example, when considering the domain of assessing mental state, it is important that the database allows both a description of mental state and records whether the assessment has been carried out. It is probably too difficult to have separate fields for each aspect of the mental state examination, so the ability to add free text will be important when providing a good description of the mental state for the accessible clinical database. In addition to free text, it may be possible to add brief categories, of which only one covering the major issue could be selected (e.g. well, depressed, psychotic).

It is also possible to code for whether the mental state examination has been carried out or not, so that the process is recorded and one is able to determine the proportion of patients in a given period without an examination (needs assessment or audit). Perhaps more importantly it is possible to obtain the names of those not receiving a mental state examination so they can be targeted for follow up.

Combining these components would produce a data entry system such as this:

Figure 6 Example data entry system

Mental state examination:	*Picking list:*	*(Choose one from below)*
		A: Mental state not examined
		B: Depressed
		C: Delusions predominant
		D: Hallucinations predominant
		E: Manic/hypomanic
		F: Negative symptoms
		G: No significant problem
		H: Other
	Free text:...	

This process could be completed for the other domains in Table 6 (p.35), which the practice has chosen to include in its database. The different general practice software systems have different methods of creating and accessing their databases or templates. Advice may be required from the appropriate help desks, but the lessons learned can be transferred to other areas of care.

Each practice-based system has its own advantages and disadvantages, but most are now based on Read codes. Read codes have not been designed for community mental health care, however, and new codes have therefore to be created. Unfortunately, as yet there is no national framework of codes, so each practice makes up its own. PCGs or health authorities working with mental health trusts would do well to work together to create a unified system.

Integrating the development of care with commissioning and contracting

Assessing needs and making decisions regarding the most appropriate arrangement for shared care introduces the issues of funding and contracting. Traditional fund-holding has rarely succeeded in significantly influencing the monopolies of local mental health providers.

Total purchasing pilots and multifunds could, in theory, have had more influence. Primary care groups have the potential to combine hospital and primary care budgets and influence primary, secondary and interface care more effectively. Currently the newly formed partnership boards, which include representatives of social and health care providers and purchasers as well as users, are likely to have more influence over the overall shape of mental health services. However, whether it is PCGs or partnership boards in control, it is highly likely that primary and secondary care will be asked to put together joint plans for areas of shared care, such as heart disease, asthma, diabetes and mental illness.

This book aims to complement these commissioning processes by encouraging practitioners and managers from both teams to meet at a practice level, engendering mutual understanding of each other's positions and concerns. Collaboration rather than contracting is seen as the key to success. The process is essentially 'joint commissioning of services by providers at a practice level'. Practices within a locality will differ and some aspects of service provision can be adapted to cater for these differences. Any agreements for change or improving quality can be substantiated in a written document, although this is not legally binding.

This agreement could, however, be used in a number of ways to compliment other more formal contracts or commissioning:

- The needs assessment and case register will provide information about the number of patients within the practice at, for example, different CPA levels. The agreement will indicate some of the criteria by which a contract can be monitored; these will add to the traditional indicators, such as finished consultant episodes or health worker contacts. Criteria could include, e.g. routes, content and timing of communication, educational input, proportion of patients whose key worker is the practice linked worker and the proportion of records with minimum data set included
- Some of the issues raised in the process may be best dealt with at a locality level, e.g. content of communication between teams. Where practices are like-minded, more can be decided at a locality level. The shared care agreements are designed to compliment and feed into agreements at a locality level, for example by allowing differing

arrangements of shared care and providing detail about the level of need in the locality.

Shifting resources to primary care

Any substantial shift to primary care for the care of patients with long-term mental health problems will require some guarantee of quality as well as a shift in resources. The primary care teams will be responsible for providing an audit of care, such as effectiveness of recall systems and health promotion provision. These can be detailed in a shared care agreement as well as in any contract with the health authority or PCG.

Funding and recognition made available to primary care teams will enable them to decide whether to increase the care provided to patients with long-term mental health problems. Changes in the law will end the division between hospital and primary care funding. It will, therefore, allow practices to bid for contracts to provide mental health care. Pilot schemes employing a system of funding by items of service or similar to health promotion payments have shown that some GPs are interested in providing more comprehensive mental health care. It is recognised that until the resources shift there will not be a substantial shift in the burden of care. This book aims to provide a basis to improve care across the primary–secondary interface in either situation. Practices that have gone through the process of establishing shared care formally and have effective systems of recall and audit will be in a better position to gain contracts for provision of community mental health care. It is more likely, though, that PCGs and partnership boards will require practices to work together with secondary services to set up joint service plans for mental illness. Experienced practices are likely to be at the heart of these agreements.

Creating a shared care agreement

A shared care agreement (SCA) is a written agreement negotiated between two parties that relates to the provision of a service they provide together. In this instance, the agreement is between the two parties in order to decide how both teams will provide services across the primary–secondary care interface. The SCAs will reflect local needs, skills, interests and resources, and specify the services to be provided complementing other forms of contracting at primary care group and health authority levels. While the process of sharing information, deciding priorities and developing services is more important than the written document itself, there are advantages to specifying details of agreements between two parties, which can be referred to at a later date. Our shared care agreements used the options in Chapters 4 and 5 as the basic template. Appendix 5 is an example.

Chapter 4

Defining the changes in detail

The joint working group is now in a position to decide on the type of shared care and to specify plans for developments to be detailed in the shared care agreement. Both teams will have met alone and decided on their preferred options. These options were identified following focus groups with professionals and the experience of developing care in 14 practices in south London. There may be other important issues that need to be addressed in different geographical settings and as new policies emerge. Chapter 7, 'Facilitators' guide to change', outlines a plan and offers ideas on how to facilitate this part of the process. The following areas can now be discussed and decisions made as to what is to be included within the agreement:

- services to be developed or maintained
- type of shared care
- definition of roles and responsibilities of primary and secondary services

Services to be developed or maintained

The choice of services to be developed between the two teams, and particularly in the practice, is an important decision, which will in some ways define the type of shared care and the responsibilities the practice takes on. Most of these services have not been shown to improve care but are recommended by experts or users' groups and are based on common sense.

The following provide a checklist of services which teams can develop, or if already in existence, improve and maintain:

- practice register
- updating mechanism for register
- joint register with CMHT team
- computer template/chronic disease card

- recall system for mental health review
- targeted recall system for mental health review (requires monitoring of processes of care)
- recall system for physical review (including health promotion)
- targeted recall system for physical review
- repeat medication system linked to reviews
- a key primary care worker for each patient not under CMHT care
- depots given by practice
- audit of care
- development of guidelines for areas of care (see Appendix 1)
- early signs education (see Appendix 1)
- creation/adaptation of a local resource directory
- setting up of a carers' group
- setting up a users' group
- obtaining of patient information leaflets for use in the practice
- annual practice needs assessment
- joint team clinical meeting
- computer-based prompts for evidence-based interventions.

Type of shared care

Available resources, current policies and the interests and preferences of the participants will define the type of shared care. This section aims to define the working relationships between the teams and professionals within the teams.

Which model of shared care will be implemented?

See pages 30–32 for more details.

Separate primary mental health care teams. These are mental health care teams funded by primary care and based in the practice, usually with external psychiatrist support.

Practice-based CPN. The CPN provides a contact point with the CMHT, provides interventions and advice, organises training, and acts as key worker to the majority of cases.

Linked liaison workers. Link workers are community mental health workers from the CMHT with limited responsibilities, primarily acting to give advice and act as a communication channel for the practice (without taking on practice cases).

Hybrid model. Community mental health workers work as part of the community team and provide advice to the linked practice but are increasingly taking on cases from the practice, as agreed by the team manager.

Shifted out-patient model. The psychiatrist conducts an out-patient clinic in the GP's surgery mostly in the absence of the GP.

Consultation–liaison model. The psychiatrist attends a primary care meeting to discuss management of patients, after which the psychiatrist sees patients, often with the GP.

Traditional one-to-one model. Over time the teams get to know each other so well that they are able to choose the most appropriate member of the other team to talk to.

Which relationships within the shared care arrangement will be dominant or which will need fostering?

- CMHW–GP
- psychiatrist–GP
- CMHW–practice nurse
- CMHW–GP–psychiatrist
- GP alone + CMHW/psychiatrist

Will the CMHT consider moving to/piloting a practice cluster-based model rather than using a geographical sector to define limits of responsibility for care?

Vignette: involving carers

LP is a 29-year-old man with schizophrenia who refused medication and would not leave his parents' small house, which he has turned into a virtual fortress, only allowing in a number of trusted friends and family. While actively psychotic, with prominent paranoid delusions, he was not a danger to others or at risk of self-harm. For both these reasons the local community team and even the local mental health organisation had stopped visiting.

Unusually, one day his father came to the surgery regarding a hernia, and stayed on a few minutes to pour his heart out about LP. It became clear that both LP's father and mother had become significantly depressed by the situation; LP's younger brother was turning increasingly to alcohol and behaving aggressively.

A visit was arranged when the father was in so that an overall assessment of the family   situation and parents' mental health could be made. LP agreed to be seen briefly from the top of the stairs, and spoke angrily. Although neither parent wanted antidepressants, they agreed for the community mental health team to become involved again on the condition that LP was not admitted to hospital. Discussion with his mother and sister suggested that they were a high 'expressed emotion' (EE) family. High EE with respect to protectiveness over involvement (in this case his mother) and disapproval (brother and sister) has been linked to a high relapse rate.

The family agreed to ongoing involvement, which included supportive counselling, further education about schizophrenia and a programme to reduce collusion with LP on non-compliance and creating a fortress house. Mrs P remained depressed and later accepted antidepressant medication, after which she showed some improvement. LP continues to refuse all medication but the family are able to operate more normally.

Definition of roles and responsibilities

Once the basic model of shared care has been defined it is important to consider how individuals and team functions fit in. Investigations into homicides and suicides involving patients with severe mental illness have often highlighted the lack of clarity of role definition across teams. This section aims to clarify the core roles and to define the responsibilities that are part of a shift towards improving quality of care.

Will the role of the psychiatrist include:

- urgent and non-urgent advice by telephone?
- availability by bleep?
- direct GP–psychiatrist out-patient referrals?
- clinics within primary care?
- discussion of difficult cases in primary care?
- regular contact with PHCT?

Will the role of attached/linked community mental health worker include:

- providing general advice on the CMHT function
- providing general advice on patients with long-term mental illness, including those not under the CMHT or within CMHT boundaries
- discussion of possible referrals? (With all new referrals allocated by team leader.)
- preferential acceptance of appropriate new referrals following discussion with team leader?
- liaising with the GP (as the responsible medical officer) to share care for more stable patients?
- initial acceptance of all (long-term mental health) referrals?
- advice and assistance to set up and maintain case register?
- having access to practice notes/computer?
- attendance at practice meetings quarterly/monthly/weekly?
- a desk space at the practice?
- providing training to the practice?

The role of primary care in the Care Programme Approach process

CPA meetings are not designed for GPs to attend and the invitations for long meetings in the midst of a busy surgery are often ignored. In spite of this, mental health workers value GPs' contributions – even if it is to inform them of a lack of contact. CPA meetings can also provide the opportunity for primary care workers to act as advocates for their patients.

Will input to the Care Programme Approach process include:

- GP attendance at CPA meeting?
- annual GP attendance at CPA meeting?
- GP written input?
- care co-ordinator/key worker contacting GP prior to CPA for discussion?
- CPA meetings to be held in the practice with GP attendance?
- CPA meetings to be held in the practice with GP attendance and physical health review by practice nurse on the same day?

Advocating Clozapine

A Care Programme Approach meeting was being held late morning nearby, so JP's GP decided to find out 'what they were like' and take the opportunity to meet the new psychiatrist. During JP's CPA it became clear that he had treatment resistant schizophrenia, causing multiple admissions and self-neglect. Having sat and listened to the proceedings, the GP recalled that Clozapine has been shown to be effective in non-responsive schizophrenia and asked if it had been tried. It had, but three years previously, and stopped immediately due to a falling blood count, which must be monitored. Treatment with Clozapine was given a second trial. GPs can act as advocates for treatment, sometimes in a more independent capacity.

Provision of full physical care

Morbidity and mortality from physical illness are increased in this group of patients and yet referrals, investigations and care of chronic illness are neglected. Will the PHCT provide:

- recall for annual health check with practice nurse (health promotion and disease prevention)?
- opportunistic health promotion?
- where appropriate, proactive investigation and referral for physical symptoms?
- liaison with key worker/carer to ensure attendance?
- advice on obtaining care from opticians, chiropodists, dentists, etc.?
- copies of significant referrals for physical problems to CMHT?

It is assumed that if the CHMT is responsible for overall mental health, then the GP would continue with responsibility for physical care and respond to need as it arose.

GPs' role in mental health care

GPs vary greatly in the extent to which they care for patients with mental illness. This reflects skills, confidence and interest as well as time constraints and historic practice. Setting up a shared care agreement provides an opportunity to look at the possible roles and how they might change. Some GPs will welcome the chance to broaden their practice in this interesting area but will feel the need for additional training. In some areas commissioning care through PCGs will provide the opportunities for being paid to look after this group. It is useful to clarify the limits of care for both the PHCT and CMHT.

For those patients *not* under the trust, will the role of GPs include:

- repeat prescribing?
- medication review?
- non-urgent changes to medication?
- Lithium monitoring and medication changes?
- recall for annual/quarterly review?
- brief risk assessment?
- mental state monitoring?
- screening for family and carer, benefits and housing needs?

Are the PHCTs willing to take on the role of caring for additional patients with long-term mental health problems? If so:

- what type of support will the CMHT provide?
- will rapid re-referral to the original trust team be possible in cases of deterioration?

Flexibility

SG was a 47-year-old woman with schizophrenia who received a depot from the CMHT; she had been stable and managing almost independently for years. She inherited £30,000, decided to move locally and bought a flat overlooking a park. Unfortunately she had crossed the geographical catchment area boundary and was due to move to a neighbouring team. Her thoughtful CPN, who knew that SG liked her family doctor, asked the practice if they would follow her up. They reached a special agreement that a CPN in the new team would give the monthly depot, but otherwise her mental health care was co-ordinated by her GP.

Core community mental health activities

The teams need to clarify for each patient whether the core activities are the responsibility of the practice or the CMHT. For each patient these activities may be divided if care is shared. Core activities might include:

- screening for mental health needs
- mental state monitoring
- medication review
- non-urgent medication changes
- Lithium and Carbamazepine bloods and associated medication changes
- prescribing repeat medication
- depot administration.

How will these responsibilities be recorded?

- on chronic disease cards?
- on shared care cards?

- in communications to and from the CMHT?
- on a computer template?
- within the trust records?
- within CMHT records?

Decisions made after working through this Chapter will fundamentally affect the type of care being provided for patients with LTMI in general practice. This care may well differ significantly from practice to practice. In order to ensure a high level of co-ordination between the PHCT and CMHT, good channels of communication are essential, and their development is described in Chapter 6.

Chapter 5

Delivering and sustaining change

This Chapter outlines the important process of making and supporting the changes in clinical practice necessary to ensure that patients receive better quality care. Particular emphasis is placed on the need to invest in training, and having efficient and assertive management processes.

Redraft and sign the shared care agreement

At this stage, the joint working group should be able to agree a document detailing all the areas and developments to be included in the agreement. This could then be circulated to all members of the two teams to ensure wider agreement and dissemination. An additional or first joint working clinical meeting might be a useful vehicle to launch the work on LTMI (see p.12).

Once agreement has been obtained by all parties concerned, the joint working group should be able to sign the agreement and set its contents in motion. It may be that teams will agree to implement the agreement for one year, evaluate and then possibly renegotiate the terms.

Setting realistic objectives

It is also helpful to decide which services should be developed/prioritised over a particular timescale, for example per year. This target setting will make the process more manageable and easier to refine.

It is suggested that each objective is 'SMART':
  S pecific
  M easurable
  A chievable
  R elevant
  T imebound

While some changes will produce early results, it is anticipated that others will take more than a year. It may be useful to look at existing systems for chronic disease management within the practice in order to replicate current procedures for maintaining registers and organising recall.

Set up a plan for each objective

1   Choose a co-ordinator responsible for planning and delivery of completed development
2   Consider barriers to change and how to overcome them
3   Break down objective into defined tasks
4   Set deadlines for completion of each task
5   List resources required (clinician time, manager time, administration/secretarial time, external expertise, advice from CMHT, examples of good practice, capital expenditure (if any))
6   Plan training for individuals involved
7   Monitor initial quality of work
8   Monitor progress (weekly/fortnightly)
9   Report back to joint working group/practice.

Saving time by combining work for a needs assessment and audit

Table 6 (p.36) details the data on patients that could be available at consultations and can also be used for audits or needs assessment. It might be kept as a paper copy, for example as a chronic illness card, or on a computerised template. The last section includes data that may be added on a routine basis, during ongoing care and perhaps extracted from letters and summaries coming from secondary care.

There is considerable overlap between the data requirements of audit and needs assessment. When setting up a register, it is possible to carry out an initial quantitative needs assessment for the practice and an audit. The process of going through each set of notes can be time consuming and it is sensible if possible to use the opportunity of reviewing the notes, to make decisions about care (e.g. who does Lithium monitoring?) as well as to flag up further data required. The suggestions below assume that the work of creating a register, choosing codes and developing a computer database or chronic disease card have been completed.

If a practice wishes to combine these activities it is suggested that a series of tasks for each patient are completed together:

- assign a diagnosis (or more than one) from the list allowed for constructing the register
- collect the data for each patient from practice records and correspondence: add to chronic disease card or computer template
- complete audit/needs assessment form (Appendix 4), unless a computerised audit has been set up
- make any clinical/organisational decisions for each patient

The work involved is not inconsiderable and can be tackled in a number of different ways. Some doctors will want to do this work themselves. Practices with experienced data inputers or summarisers could use these people to do the bulk of the work, ensuring that the quality is checked at the start and that they have access to medical advice at the end of each session. Alternatively, if the practice invites this group of patients for a review of physical or mental health the work can be done at that time of review spread over several months.

Planning training for PHCT and CMHT members

Training for members of the PCHT and CMHT can help develop skills for shared care. Training could be based on local need, individual interests and available options, according to personal learning plan principles.

Link workers may benefit from training in the following areas:

- working alone in a culture that may at times be hostile
- working to help solve problems regarding patients for whom they are not the care co-ordinator
- giving advice and making decisions following a more limited mental health assessment
- understanding the structure and function of primary care
- being a representative of the community mental health team.

GPs and practice nurses have a variety of learning needs:

- carrying out mental state examinations
- screening for a variety of psychosocial needs
- having a basic understanding of long-term mental illness (for nurses)
- to be updated on management of psychosis and severe depression
- setting up and running the systems required to keep a register and recall patients.

Practices are advised to assess both the individual and team skills and knowledge deficits, related to areas of service provision and development within the shared care agreement for LTMI. With experience and ongoing training, PHCTs can provide:

- mental health assessments, overall management and use of anti-psychotic medication for people with severe mental health problems
- recognition and management of depression and stress, mental state assessment, administration and review of medication by non-GP members
- recognition and prevention of depression in young mothers/children.

Teams may also consider the following:

- development of a training calendar and invitation of guest speakers
- the allocation of time for staff training
- setting up a training budget
- the supervision of staff
- informal and formal team support
- supportive feedback on performance
- availability of a senior member of staff for advice in crisis situations
- identifying training deficits among team members
- integrating practice and individual learning needs into personal learning plans.

Training can take the form of:

- local PGEA approved courses
- specially organised seminars/educational afternoons
- a series of 'consultation liaison' sessions with a local psychiatrist or

senior CPN
- reading material and videos
- joint training initiatives by either team
- 'shadowing' members of the other team.

In order to help encourage changes to clinical practice, certain interventions may be more effective than others; these include face-to-face instruction, computer prompts and peer review with practice visits.

The following example questionnaire can be adapted by teams and used to assess the training needs of all team members.

Figure 7 Assessment of training needs: example questionnaire

Name ....

Job Title ....

We are looking at the training needs of the whole primary care team/community mental health team in mental health. Please could you complete the following brief questions to help assess your needs and plan appropriate training.

Are you interested in further mental health training to suit your needs?

YES/NO

If yes, please go to question 1.

If no, why not?

....

....

1. What are your preferred methods of learning? Please tick as many as you like.

Reading ☐

Shadow/sit in clinics with specialist nurse or doctor ☐

Lectures ☐

Videos ☐

Problem/patient-based discussion ☐

Group work ☐

Other ....

2. Where would be your preferred location of training?

....

....

3. Which of the following areas would you like more training in, first with your existing work load, and second if you were to see more long-term mental health problems?

	Existing Work load	More Mental Health Problems Seen
Mental state exam (psychosis)	☐	☐
Assessing suicide risk/depression	☐	☐
Prescribing anti-psychotics	☐	☐
Monitoring medication	☐	☐
Mental Health Acts/sections	☐	☐
Resistant/chronic depression	☐	☐
Assessing overall needs of patients	☐	☐
Dealing with violent or aggressive patients	☐	☐
Definition of roles and responsibilities of PHCT/CMHT	☐	☐
Communication skills Family intervention	☐	☐

Monitoring and evaluation of shared care

Auditing care

Monitoring progress can be useful to ensure that successes are celebrated and failures are addressed. Data collection can be time consuming, but once data is being efficiently captured and organised on a computerised template it is relatively easy on most systems to set up audits to monitor progress and stimulate discussion about which areas of care need further improvement. The following audits may be carried out using the available data:

- the quality of data collection (e.g. the percentage of patients on the register with no record of self-harm, risk status or the number of patients on the practice register with psychotic diagnoses that are not on the recommended list of Read codes)
- processes of care (e.g. the number of patients who had had a mental state or physical examination completed)
- outputs of care (e.g. the number of patients with normal blood pressure or normal Lithium level).

Appendix 4 gives further ideas for data collection. In addition more qualitative *critical incident audits* could be carried out. These could involve discussions of suicides, overdoses, sections, violence or simply relapses, in order to learn how systems may be improved.

Evaluating the development of shared care

The two teams will need a mechanism for evaluating and improving the developments agreed on. This could take the form of:

- regular practice/CMHT reviews
- monitoring of agreed developments
- dissemination of a quarterly/annual report to both teams on progress
- annual review of the shared care agreement, considering successes and problems, the political and economic environment and assessment and decision-making procedures.

Chapter 6

Improving communication

Good quality communication between professionals is increasingly important as teams become more specialised, patients' expectations rise and turn-over of staff and patients increases. Research and audits have repeatedly demonstrated that communication between general practices and mental health professionals is often felt to be unsatisfactory, particularly with respect to content. While it is possible to develop systems through a practice-based intervention as described in the previous Chapters, it is unlikely that major changes to the way the secondary services provide information to primary care can be achieved in this way. Furthermore, the community-based mental health staff often have problems obtaining sufficient and timely information from their hospital counterparts.

This Chapter therefore assumes that the changes and improvements being discussed are occurring at a trust or primary care group (PCG) wide level. It is therefore suggested that a meeting should be arranged between these two bodies ensuring adequate grass roots representation from primary care workers and community and hospital mental health workers. The following areas could be addressed:

- team contact details
- communication content
- use of information technology

It is recommended that a small working group draws up recommendations to be discussed by the larger group, before sending out to all concerned for consultation.

Team contact details and methods of communication

Easy access to named professionals in other teams by telephone, fax or email can make small yet important tasks and communications easier to achieve. If possible there should be a system for updating information regularly. The details outlined on pages 16–17 provide an example of the information that might be made available to collaborating teams across the PCG. Individual community mental health teams may vary or there may be a trust policy for preferred methods of contact. Optimising the balance of face-to-face, telephone and written communication is a further objective.

How will contact routinely be made with the CMHTs?

- with individual teams, e.g. case management, assessment and treatment or rehabilitation?
- via a single central telephone number?
- through the link worker?
- directly with the key worker or consultant psychiatrist?

How will urgent referrals be made to CMHTs?

- to the crisis team or direct to psychiatrists for emergency assessments?
- to the key worker, psychiatrist or link worker for urgent problems of current clients?
- to the link worker, assessment and treatment team or duty desk for new cases?

Communication content

Poor communication between the PHCT and CMHT causes problems for the effective delivery of mental health care. To communicate effectively, certain information is required in letters and reports by both services. An optimum level of communication needs to be reached to ensure that the essentials are transferred without wasting valuable time and effort. The following is a relatively exhaustive list of the possible contents of communication additional to basic clinical details, which are normally well documented:

Information required by the CMHT in referral letters

- social and family background of patient
- explicit reason for referral
- responsibilities that the GP is willing to take on

- urgency of case (in weeks)
- risk of harm to self or others
- medication and therapies received
- telephone number of patient

It should be confirmed whether the CMHT requires a referral form to be completed, or if it is sufficient to include the above information in a letter.

Information required by the PHCT in assessment, follow up and discharge letters

The information required will vary depending on whether the assessment is at discharge from hospital, on first contact or at routine follow up. Table 9 details the type of data that may be useful to primary care, particularly as more practices and CMHTs develop computer databases. The following information, which is less easy to categorise and code, may also be useful:

- current level of risk of harm, i.e. suicide, self-neglect, violence
- knowledge of patient and relatives/carers of the patient's condition
- predicted course of condition and its effect on the patient's lifestyle
- management plan, including review date
- anticipated roles of CMHT and PHCT
- mental state on discharge
- expected early signs of relapse and action to take.

Table 9 Data input for long-term mental illness: transfer to primary care

Socio-demographic data
Name
Address, telephone no.
Sex, date of birth
Marital status: *married, single, separated, widowed, divorced*
Ethnicity:
Housing type: *council, housing association, rented, owned, hostel, no fixed abode*
Home situation: *lives alone – with help, lives alone – no help, lives with partner, lives with family, single parent*
Number of children/dependants
Next of kin/address/telephone no.
Neighbour/main carer/address/telephone no

Accumulated clinical data
Diagnosis
Date of diagnosis
Previous Mental Health Act section: *types and dates*
History of deliberate self-harm
History of harm to others
Substance misuse: *alcohol, opiates, benzodiazepines, other*
Specific indicators of relapse
Specific crisis response
CPA level: *1, 2, 3, not specified; date*
Supervision register: *Y/N; date*
Section 117: *date*

Service contact
CMHT: name
Psychiatrist
CPN
Care co-ordinator/key worker
Social worker
Housing worker
Other involved agency 1: telephone no.
Involved agency 2: telephone no.
Involved agency 3: telephone no.

Sharing of care
Main care: *CMHT, GP, GP–CMHW, Psychiatrist–GP, CMHT–GP (first partner responsible for overall needs assessment, recall, if required, mental state monitoring, risk assessment, organising CPAs, medication review and non-urgent changes to medication)*

Other responsibilities that may reside with the second partner in shared care:
- Lithium bloods
- Lithium medication changes
- repeat prescribing
- depot administration and recall

Recall policy
Frequency of reviews
Date of next review

Data from latest contact
Current mental state
Current risk of deliberate self-harm
Current risk of harm to others
Risk of self-neglect
Current medication reviewed: *Y/N with free text compliance*
Lithium levels sent, or actual level
Depot given: *date*
Accommodation needs
Needs for activities of daily living
Leisure/activities needs
Carer/family issues
Benefits reviewed: *date and outcome*
Physical care needs or concerns for PHCT to address

Information from primary care consultations and community contacts

Currently it is not traditional for information from primary care contacts or community mental health contacts to be passed on. While it may not be necessary for all contacts to be communicated, the following may be considered for patients whose care is shared:

- faxed outcome of urgent/emergency assessments regardless of outcome
- communication to secondary services of significant contacts in primary care
- copies of referrals to acute hospitals for physical care
- six-monthly or annual reviews of care provided by community teams in addition to CPA reports.

Communication during time of hospitalisation

As in-patient stays become shorter, there are more early readmissions and hospital stays are also broken by phased discharges. It is important for hospital wards to provide timely information to both primary care and community-based colleagues, e.g.:

- fax of admission details to the PHCT and CMHT
- invitation to the practice to be involved in discharge planning
- faxed information to the practice and CMHT regarding staged discharges and leave
- details to be faxed on the day of discharge
- essential details, including roles, to be clear and at the head of the discharge summary.

Shared care records and crisis cards

Shared care records come in a number of guises and have been used successfully in a small number of settings and districts. They may be primarily for patients or designed to inform other professionals about the patients' details of diagnosis, medication and appointments. They have obvious advantages, but there is resistance to developing them from both users and professionals. Crisis cards have been developed to focus on the individual needs of patients during a crisis, from their preferred medication to who will look after the cat. The patient holds them but the information is also available on an electronic database that may be accessed at a variety of locations. This can in turn be linked to a district wide register. Both shared care records and crisis cards require substantial planning and co-ordinated implementation.

Standards of communication and criteria for referral

PCGs may wish to set standards for both primary and secondary services to adhere to. For example:

- agreeing a time period for sending/receiving assessment, review and referral letters
- agreeing deadlines for responding to referrals
- agreeing criteria for referral and discharge

- setting out a procedure for refused referrals.

Setting standards and criteria has advantages but may risk precipitating confrontation rather than close collaboration. It is essential that acceptable frameworks for dealing with issues that arise are established. In particular, practices will differ in their level of skills for dealing with this group of patients and therefore it may be appropriate to link any feedback to educational objectives. Furthermore, it may be appropriate for criteria for referral to differ from practice to practice, dependent on the levels of co-operation, skills and details of practice-based shared care agreements.

Using information technology to improve communication

There is now a common vision amongst practitioners with interests in shared care and using IT effectively, to use the NHS Net to transfer core information across the primary–secondary interface. These ideas have not been fully tested and there is no substantive forum for developing the vision into a cohesive workable programme, particularly in the area of LTMI. Nevertheless, the technology now exists for transfer of patient information associated with new NHS numbers in order to allow:

- direct informing of practice databases by secondary care information
- updating of district or regional registers by primary care
- availability of IT-based crisis plans for all out-of-hours contacts
- accessibility of shared patient databases from primary and secondary care
- carrying out needs assessments across the interface
- shared performance indicators and targets.

In addition to the changes in attitudes and culture that primary care groups may bring, these potentially valuable contributions to improving quality will require close joint working between managers and practitioners in primary and secondary care to:

- agree useful diagnostic groupings
- agree how key information will be coded
- pilot methods of transferring information to and from the variety of

primary care IT systems
- agree inclusion criteria for different levels of register
- agree access to shared databases

Whilst the full development of these systems will have to wait, much useful work can be done now to establish a mutually acceptable language and series of codes, which can be used with current paper systems.

Chapter 7

Facilitators' guide to change

This Chapter provides a theoretical and practical approach to the role of the facilitator in the development of the shared care process between primary health care teams and community mental health teams outlined in this book. In addition, we have included plans for the joint working group meetings and some examples from experience. It should prove useful both to official facilitators and to readers who take on the role by default, having initially been asked to co-ordinate or chair the meetings.

The need for facilitation

General practices and community mental health teams both deal with patients with long-term mental illness who live in the community. However, their origins, professions and cultures of teamwork are very different. Community mental health teams were established as a direct result of moving patients with long-term mental illness into the community and are now the vehicle for provision of community-based services in most parts of the country. With all the changes within the NHS affecting both primary and secondary care, it seems that both general practices and community mental health teams will be here to stay. Bringing these two teams together will provide a basis for an efficient primary–secondary interface by:

- meeting face-to-face
- building trust
- sharing ideas
- interacting creatively
- improving communication
- clarifying responsibilities.

The ultimate aim of bringing the two teams together is to improve the care of patients with long-term mental illness; it will be necessary to enhance the skills and confidence of primary care workers and link workers to take on new roles and create effective new systems of care.

This kind of interaction at the primary–secondary interface is new to many involved, and can result in anxiety and suspicion. With increased pressure in primary care resulting from early discharges, some GPs are keen to protect themselves from additional work. Similarly, community mental health teams are setting thresholds for the type of patient they are willing to care for, in order to control work load. These initiatives tend to set up barriers between teams rather than encourage joint working. To counter this, the joint working group process aims to build trust so that responsibilities can be shared in an efficient and patient-centred way:

- community mental health teams might have the confidence to discharge patients back into primary care; general practices will begin to trust that when patients have been discharged, they can get early support from the community teams rather than always going through inefficient referral and assessment procedures
- community mental health teams might provide informal advice and input regarding patients who are not their responsibility, which may result in less referrals for expensive and time consuming assessments
- joint working may result in more appropriate direct referrals to the member of the community mental health team best placed to help.

In the future, setting up joint working or defining shared care may become a requirement under the guise of clinical governance or new primary care groups. However, there are currently few incentives to encourage the kind of changes laid out in this book.

Developing the process of joint working is a complex task, which will touch sensitivities and take time. The research project that developed the processes described in this book used a system of facilitation and also gave participants' practices small financial incentives.

The entire process of facilitating the joint working groups, including initial training and follow up, will take a facilitator perhaps half a day per week per practice. Practices might receive about £2000 for participation and development of a register. This one-off cost of £50–£60 per patient in a medium-to-large inner city practice compares favourably with some modern anti-psychotic medications.

Having a facilitator provides many advantages:

- someone whose main role is to bring the teams together
- someone with skills in handling meetings
- someone, as an outsider, who can defuse tensions and provide objectivity
- someone with time to manage the process of joint decision making
- someone who can push the process forward to implement change.

Facilitation: a theoretical framework

This section describes a model of facilitation, which can be used as a theoretical framework for running joint working groups. This model is based on Rogers' seminal work, *Freedom To Learn*. The joint working groups should be based on the philosophy of valuing everyone's views and highlighting the skills and experience that the different group members can offer.

The role of the facilitator

- the facilitator is first concerned with establishing a climate of trust
- the facilitator encourages the use of ground rules
- the facilitator seeks clarification of each members' aims and tolerates a diversity of skills within the group
- the facilitator relies on the motivation of each member to pursue their own aims, which are significant only to themselves
- the facilitator acts in a flexible way, as a resource to the group
- the facilitator recognises and accepts group members' thoughts and feelings, giving due weight to each
- the facilitator becomes a participant member as the group develops
- the facilitator shares his or her own thoughts and feelings with the group
- the facilitator is alert to tensions and conflicts in the group, which can be utilised as learning resources
- the facilitator is aware of and accepts his or her strengths and weaknesses as a facilitator and as a resource

Managing the group discussion

The contributions made by all individuals in the group discussions need to be treated with respect. The facilitator should:

- encourage one person to speak at a time
- not belittle what people are saying (and be aware of non-verbal behaviour)
- bring everybody in
- build on suggestions and reflect other contributions
- offer support and agreement when appropriate
- confront unhelpful members on the basis of ground rules
- deflect unpleasantness through peer pressure
- use humour
- reframe by looking at different perspectives
- above all, be positive.

Confidentiality

There is a need for confidentiality in the joint working groups. Both facilitators and group members can easily assume that there is a common level of understanding that confidentiality will be underpinning the process, but this is not always the case. It is useful if the facilitator briefly addresses the issue of confidentiality at the beginning of the group, perhaps when the ground rules are being laid down. One definition of confidentiality is, 'keeping trust with others by not divulging personal information about them unless granted permission.' (Richard Nelson James).

What roles will a good chairperson adopt?

- the consensus builder
- the sympathetic listener
- the organiser/manager
- the arbitrator
- the leader
- the time keeper
- the summariser/secretary

Group members' experience of facilitation

It is likely that the nature of a group will change depending on the overall aims of the group and on individual members' characteristics and learning styles. The facilitator will need to acknowledge that members of the joint working group will often start from different points and will develop their contribution and ideas, and assimilate information at different speeds. We have outlined a theoretical model, which may be useful in understanding how people work, learn and behave within a group.

This model is based on David Kolb's theory (*Experiential Learning*, 1984) that people learn from experience in terms of a cycle with four clear stages: concrete experience, reflective observation, abstract conceptualism and active experimentation.

Figure 8

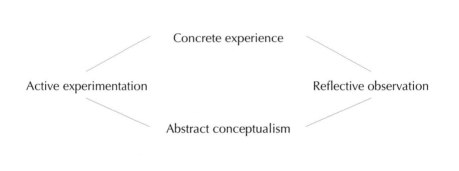

Honey and Mumford (*Manual of Learning Styles*, 1986) have used Kolb's research as a basis for suggesting that people have individual learning preferences that fit with different stages of the cycle:

1 **Activists** learn well from immediate experience. They tend to be open-minded and enthusiastic about anything new, although they become bored with longer-term consolidation. They often act first and think afterwards. Brainstorming solves problems. Activists like to be the centre of activity.

2   **Reflectors** learn best by having time to think back to experiences. They are thorough, collecting information from all sources, and like to complete this process before coming to a decision. On the whole they are cautious, thoughtful people who tend to take a back seat, enjoying seeing other people in action. They naturally tend to adopt a low profile.

3   **Theorists** learn by logical, abstract thought. They tend to be perfectionists and like to be able to fit information into a structure. Their behaviour is likely to be detached and analytical, they feel uncomfortable with emotional and subjective judgements.

4   **Pragmatists** learn by trying out new ideas to see if they work. Usually they are full of ideas, and they will take every opportunity to experiment, to see if the ideas work. They like to get on with things quickly and are likely to be impatient. They enjoy challenges and are essentially down to earth, practical people who enjoy problem solving.

Facilitation of the joint working groups

Preparation before the meetings

It is recommended that each member of the JWG has a copy of this book, to enable full participation and understanding. The following preparation is recommended before the meetings, which are likely to take the form of three one-and-a-half hour sessions:

- book all the meetings at least one month in advance
- ensure the meeting place is acceptable to all concerned
- request that the participants read all necessary information before the meeting
- circulate the minutes of the preceding meeting two weeks before the next meeting.

Just before holding a meeting

- be prepared and organise an agenda in good time before the meeting
- find out about the two teams and participants during informal telephone conversations when planning dates; it also helps to meet key members before the meeting

- arrive early and set up the meeting room before others turn up
- be aware of the physical environment, e.g. the layout of the room. Avoid confrontational styles of seating
- start on time
- consider the issues specific to these two teams
- plan to present each item and issue clearly

Plans for the joint working groups

The following plans were used by the facilitators working with the joint working groups in south London. They can and should be adapted according to the needs of the group. The joint working group may complete the work in three or four meetings. The agenda of each meeting can start from where the last meeting finished, following the lists below. Sometimes, by mutual agreement, the groups have met four or even five times.

A plan for the first joint working group

Beforehand, send a brief agenda, with the time and place of the meeting and a request to read Chapters 1 and 2 of this book.

Part 1: introductions

- introduction of facilitator and people attending; agreement of time to end meeting
- agreement on ground rules: mutual respect, one person talking at a time, open constructive criticism of current services (present these rather than spending too long developing them)
- what is the project about?
- description of overall aims and objectives
- introduction of the purpose of the joint working group meetings
- brief explanation of the facilitator role (and perhaps apologise in advance for redirecting conversations in order to keep to time)

Part 2: visions for change

This part provides an opportunity for differing agendas to emerge:

- group discussion about views on current service provision and ideas for change
- group discussion about potential barriers to success. (This discussion can be preceded by a few minutes' silence while participants are asked to consider the ambitions they have as teams and individuals for the project; they can then be asked specifically to present their ideas and respond to each other in turn rather than to the facilitator. This is a useful technique for getting the group to work together as a team and takes the pressure off the facilitator, who might consider drawing their chair back from the group and taking notes with minimal intervention to keep things on track.)

Part 3: the basics

- discussion to find a working definition of long-term mental illness (referring to page 11 of this book)
- consideration of the needs and priorities of patients under the care of the practice and the community mental health team (see Chapter 2)
- exchange of information about current working practices and services

Part 4: finishing up

- housekeeping activity to check that joint working group members' names and contact details are correct, and who will be attending the next meeting
- clarification of information needs and process of gathering/swapping information
- action plan – who will do what by when?
- set agenda for future meetings
- request that key members of each team meet separately to decide their preferences for the options laid out in Chapters 3 and 4, which should be read
- set date, time and place of future meeting(s) (perhaps swapping venues)
- circulate minutes and record of follow-up actions

Joint working groups two and three: deciding on future care

This section deals with the work of ensuring that decisions are made to cover the various aspects of a shared care agreement and the development of services. People within the group will be working at different speeds so the facilitator may need to revisit earlier concepts. They will need to be sensitive to, and not surprised by, sudden changes in mood within the group. It is quite understandable that when some of the work load implications are recognised there will be backtracking on both sides. At these times it may be necessary for the facilitator to take on a proactive role to gently explain the advantages of new options rather than accepting the status quo; on the other hand, the final decisions have to be those of the group or the team concerned. The facilitator can therefore take on the role of the persuader but not the decision-maker; these moments of persuasion should be limited or the teams will feel bullied and reject the process outright.

A complex new area of care is being discussed and one decision will have further implications. For example, the type of patients involved will have an effect on the construction of a register and the changes in the services and practice will determine the functions of the register. There will therefore be times when decisions appear to have been made but need to be revisited and clarified or adapted.

A plan for the second joint working group meeting

Part 1: reviewing the situation

- introduction of new members
- reflections on the previous meeting
- issues arising from the minutes of the previous meeting(s)
- ensuring that the details of each team have been exchanged
- reaffirming the type of patients who will be involved
- consideration of any work on needs assessment that has been done, e.g. numbers of patients with psychosis found on practice computer search

Part 2: decision time (follow Chapters 4, 5 and 6)

- consideration of the possible functions of the register (reflection on the group's visions)
- consideration of the options of the shared care model
- consideration of the role of the link worker
- consideration of the role of the psychiatrist

(And continuing to work through Chapters 4, 5 and parts of 6.)

Part 3: ending

- give ten minutes to wind each meeting up
- confirm date of next meeting and action points to be carried out, particularly regarding the register, which may be constructed in parallel with the group

Completing the third (and fourth) meetings of the joint working group

- ensure that specific achievable developments are decided on
- agree dates to achieve these by, and people to co-ordinate (see Chapter 6)
- agree on any support required for constructing the register
- agree on any training required
- agree on how to proceed with the shared care agreement
- agree on a date for a review meeting: three months has been found useful

Trouble shooting

When the theory of facilitation is applied to practice it may not seem easy to perform the various skills and roles that are required. This can be due to a number of issues that will affect your ability and role of facilitator. As a facilitator you cannot always control the way the discussion progresses, for example if there are a number of confident and dominant characters in your group you may need to exercise more control and assert your role of facilitator within the group. Try to keep your aims clear and give yourself space to think when you feel you are losing control. We have outlined a number of issues that may arise unexpectedly:

Hierarchical conflict. This may manifest itself in a situation where the more powerful people in the group tend to dominate the discussion and others who may not be so senior are ignored or left out of the discussion altogether. Carefully ensure all are heard but do not antagonise the decision-makers!

Internal conflict. Members of the joint working group who work with each other may not get along. This may have the effect of people talking down to, or over, others. Try to look for and reflect any agreement rather than dwelling on differences.

Backtracking. At points in the group discussions people may decide that they do not wish to pursue an idea or would like to have more time to deliberate an issue. This may have a range of effects on a group: the group may become demotivated and despondent or frustrated and annoyed that things are not going as planned. It may be worth contacting individuals outside the group to discuss specific issues.

Running out of time. Meetings can generate enthusiasm and conflict, both of which take up valuable time. When you start running late negotiate with the group whether an additional meeting or minutes at the end are acceptable. If not, be aware of parts of the process that can be cut out to ensure you finish on time.

Lateness and absence. If members of the group are late or absent this may have an effect on the group dynamics. Remember this includes you as a facilitator. If someone clearly cannot or will not attend try to involve them outside of the meetings as they may still have valuable contributions or be important in ratifying any decisions.

Personal or team agendas. There will almost certainly be a number of group or personal agendas operating within a group which are not relevant to the aims and purpose of the group. It is worth trying to uncover some of these agendas before the group meeting takes place.

Contrariness and resistance. Individuals or the group will express doubt and outright opposition to proposals you put forward. Remember that you as the facilitator are doing them a favour by being there. Let them express dissent, it is their right and their time. More importantly it is their future not yours: they must make the decisions. It can be useful to reframe resistance to your proposals as a decision about service development, which they as a team or group have to make.

Disinterest. Research suggests a lack of willingness on the part of GPs to work with patients with long-term mental illness. Our selected groups did not usually display a lack of interest but when it occurs it is important to find those areas where there is a preference to work, and to look for overlapping agendas with the mental health teams. This could involve looking in more detail at physical care or developing clear guidelines on referral rather than shared care.

The facilitator's state of mind. Your composure and ability to conduct the meeting will be affected if things have not gone to plan, if you do not feel well, if people have cancelled or you have turned up late to start a meeting. It is useful to build in time for mutual support with other facilitators or work colleagues, if possible away from the participants. Set a time for debriefing after the workshop. We found it useful for one person with a good understanding of both primary and mental health care to act formally as a discussant; the debriefing would include a discussion of options available for the next meeting.

Some common issues discussed in detail

What kind of register?

It has been recommended for many years now that primary health care teams should have a register of patients with long-term mental illness. This is not based on good evidence but is a recommendation of experts and has not yet been shown to achieve improvements in care or health outcome. Indeed, this is true for all the possible specific functions of the register. This means that decisions will be based more on goodwill and on personal and group preferences and any financial rewards associated with the construction of the register. As a facilitator it is important to be aware of how registers can work, for example by constructing box files similar to the traditional asthma, hypertension and diabetes registers used by GPs and practice nurses. It is also useful to understand how computerised registers linked to templates of data offer the possibility of an updateable database, ongoing needs assessments, audits and recall systems. It is important to understand the need for data being categorised when using these systems. Consideration may also be given to systems already in place in the practice and community team, and any local agreements regarding the types of data that may be used in needs assessment or quality review. As a facilitator it would be useful to understand not only the practices' systems but also their skills and preferences. It may be better to opt for a box file system of register that is going to be successful than pretend that a fully operational computerised register can be implemented without the necessary skills.

Traditional values

In one practice the community mental health team started with a hard line on the trust policy for link workers who were to work primarily at a means of communication. The GPs stated that if they were unable to have a practice-based CPN they would not want a link worker at all. They would prefer to re-establish the kind of traditional one-to-one communications they had had several years ago when teams were more stable and relationships had been built up. The mental health team did not want to encourage any model with a resemblance to practice-based CPNs. It required relatively forceful facilitation to explain and reword the concept of a link worker who would be gradually allocated more patients for a practice (hybrid model), but would not upset the balance of work load between community mental health workers. Eventually it was seen by the practice that link workers could be useful for discussing cases not currently under the responsibility of secondary services. Furthermore, the concept of the traditional one-to-one approach was also emphasised within the shared care agreement. The details of key members of each team were clearly laid out in the agreement.

Models of shared care and the role of the link worker

This topic often generates the most discussion and disagreement. The practices with an interest in mental health often hark back to the days of attached CPNs and would like to follow the practice-based CPN model. Mental health trusts, following Government guidance, may have a policy of withdrawing CPNs from practice and offering a link worker as a means of communication. Often the role of the facilitator has had to be one of persuasion and information at this stage: a typical discussion may involve the facilitator explaining the benefits of having a link worker who is able to give advice about patients who are not formally under the trust. This will give GPs the confidence that they can manage some of these patients more effectively. The trust in turn may see advantages in a reduction in the numbers of formal referrals.

Many community mental health teams will reject the idea of an attached community mental health worker who receives referrals direct from GPs. Discussion about the hybrid model developed in south-east London and based on the experience of attached social workers may be needed. It is possible to preferentially allocate patients to the link worker when they come from the same practice in order to start building a more meaningful relationship based on shared clinical cases. As long as the team leader still retains the co-ordinating role for the work load of all community mental health workers it is possible to ensure that the team does not have a net increased work load.

The third contentious area is that of the primary health care team taking on more responsibility for managing patients with long-term mental illness. The evidence suggests that it is likely that there are considerable numbers of patients who, although having psychotic illnesses, are not being cared for by a specialist mental health team. In addition there are many people with severe continuing or recurrent depression who are not engaged with services. Sometimes this is appropriate but at other times it is by default.

When the members of the joint working group recognise this, both the primary health care team and the community mental health team members see an increase of work load looming. They understandably consider backtracking on commitments to identify and care for this group. Until general practices start competing with community trusts (or putting in joint bids) for community mental health care contracts there is little money available for GPs to take on the responsibility of caring fully for these patients.

One aim is for there to be at least some kind of proactive review with an assessment of mental state, a medication review and a very basic screening for psychosocial problems. This becomes a possibility if the practice believes it has the backup of the community mental health team to deal with any unmet needs as they arise. It is also useful to look at the numbers involved, which will not be great for any one practice. For example, if a practice identifies 40 patients with a psychotic illness perhaps only ten will not be under the care of the trust and still be requiring this kind of care.

The varied role of the psychiatrist

Psychiatrists, like GPs and other health professionals, have different preferences and have adopted varied roles within the community mental health team. Some are central to the management of the teams while others have less influence and no line management functions, focusing on in- and out-patient work.

The joint working groups provided an opportunity for reappraisal of these roles but rather than stimulating change they tended to make the current role more explicit. One GP was surprised to hear that the psychiatrist had virtually abandoned out-patient work but acted as a key member of the community mental health team providing skills in diagnosis, risk management and medication. This role was often in an advisory capacity with far less direct contact with patients. Another psychiatrist, while yearning to do 'true community psychiatry' and see patients in general practices, was unable to make time, pulled by other in- and out-patient commitments. The joint working groups and the shared care agreements made it easier for the primary health care team to understand how the psychiatrists now worked.

Supporting and sustaining change

When the joint working groups have finished there will normally be a period of about three months between the end of the last working group and the review meeting. During this time the teams will need to begin some of the work agreed during the joint working groups, such as setting up a practice register or the link worker attending practice meetings.

At this stage the role of the facilitator will change and will be mainly consultative and supportive. The role will depend to some extent on the needs and skills of the practices and community mental health teams concerned but will almost certainly include:

- providing positive feedback to practices
- letting everyone know the extent and limits of the support you can offer
- supporting construction of the register
- completion and dissemination of the shared care agreement
- providing information
- motivating the practices and community mental health team
- motivating the facilitators by debriefing with other facilitation team members.

It has been found that extra input by the facilitator at this stage is useful where practices have little support or the systems must be put in place before implementing the work. Short meetings with practice members or community mental health team members have been found to be a good way of motivating and supporting team members who are not equipped with the necessary skills to be able to carry out the work. While a facilitator may not be familiar with the intricacies of a particular practice-based IT system, they may be able to guide practitioners to the help they need. Often at this point it may be worth enrolling the support of the practice manager who may not have attended the more clinically-orientated discussions. An understanding of audit is another useful skill that can be passed on to some practitioners. Facilitators involved in developing practices' capabilities and systems have testified about the need to improve these basic skills and systems within practices.

Ending contact with the team

There should be an explicit contract at the start (which may be renegotiated) for how long the facilitator should be involved. One year after the start, perhaps at an annual review, is a possible option for ending contact and celebrating successes. At this stage it may be useful to hand over some of the co-ordinating roles of the facilitator, to ensure any unfinished business is continued.

Conclusion

This Chapter outlines a possible model, joint working group plans and some practical advice for using the facilitation method of developing a process of shared care between community mental health teams and primary health care teams. There are, however, many different strategies for group working and facilitation and it may be that you wish to choose a different model, construct your own model or adapt the model presented in this Chapter accordingly to suit your aims.

Appendix 1

Good practice guidelines

Teams may develop good practice guidelines for the consultation, planning and review of care. The following may act as a guide, particularly for nurses involved in care of patients with mental illness.

Key facts about patients with mental illness

- 1 in 100 will suffer from schizophrenia at some time in their life
- 1 in 10 will suffer from severe depression or mania at some time in their life
- almost half lose contact with mental health services and may see only their GP
- 45 per cent have severe concurrent physical morbidity

Good practice in the consultation

There are a number of areas that can be reviewed during a consultation:

- physical status
- mental state assessment and suicide risk
- medication review and administration
- extrapyramidal side-effects/tardive dyskinesia
- patient relapse prevention strategies
- housing, social and other needs
- patient and family education and support
- review of care plan and contact with secondary services.

These can be addressed opportunistically or during a proactive review, particularly for those not under the care of the CMHT.

Table 10 Common symptoms of schizophrenia

Positive symptoms:
- hallucinations
- delusions
- agitation
- tension
- paranoia
- insomnia
- thought disorder/broadcast

Negative symptoms:
- poor grooming and hygiene
- poor social skills
- inability to experience pleasure
- limited spontaneous conversation
- poverty of speech
- blunted emotions
- little motivation

Physical health review

The following includes the areas to consider in a physical health review, which may be carried out by a GP or practice nurse:

- *circulatory:* high blood pressure, ischaemic heart disease, cerebrovascular disease
- *respiratory:* chronic bronchitis
- *obesity/underweight:* advice on diet
- *endocrine:* diabetes mellitus, thyroid disease
- *other:* chiropody, visual, dental and hearing problems
- *drug side-effects:* abnormal movements of the mouth and tongue, restlessness, stiffness, excessive salivation
- *family planning:* including cervical smear test
- *health education:* advice on smoking, alcohol intake, exercise.

Suicide risk factors

The risk of suicide is greater in people with schizophrenia, manic-depression and other psychotic disorders. Many of these contact their GP in the weeks before their death.

Table 11 Risk Factors for suicide

Personal factors:
- male
- unemployed
- single/widowed/divorced
- past suicide attempts
- recent suicide attempt

Situational factors:
- onset of an acute phase
- in-patient admission
- four weeks to three months after discharge
- discharge against medical advice
- negative family/carer attitudes

Early signs recognition

Comprehensive programmes of drug and psychosocial interventions with adults who show early signs and symptoms of schizophrenic disorders may contribute to reducing the incidence and prevalence of florid episodes of schizophrenia (Falloon *et al.*, *Journal of the Royal Society of Medicine*, 1996). These benefits are achieved by involving family practitioners, other primary care providers and the patients and significant others in the early detection of psychotic features.

Successful alliances between patients, carers and GPs can allow the recognition of symptoms that occur prior to a patient relapsing. In the event of a suspected relapse, a previously agreed plan can be implemented. The following table details the stressors and signs of relapse that patients may have, together with suggested coping strategies:

Table 12 Assorted stressors, signs of relapse and possible coping strategies for psychotic illnesses

Typical stressors	Various signs of relapse	Possible coping strategies
job loss	sleep loss	avoiding/withdrawing from situations
relationship problems	withdrawal/isolation	
financial problems	anxiety	talking to a friend
housing problems	behaviour change	sport
too much socialising	change in appetite	stimulating activity
over stimulating environ-	loss of interest in self	increasing medication
ment, e.g. pub	mood change	use of a sedative at night
bereavement	abnormal beliefs	consultation with
anniversary	hallucinations/delusions	GP/key worker
redundancy		
may be none		

Appendix 2

Prescribing and monitoring

This Appendix may be particularly useful for nurses unfamiliar with treatment decision for patients with mental illness.

Principles for prescribing anti-psychotic medication

1   Repeated monitored attempts should be made to reduce the dosage to the minimum effective level to avoid long-term side-effects
2   Anti-cholinergic medications, e.g. Procyclidine should not be routinely prescribed as they can produce tardive dyskinesia
3   Individuals can work closely with their relatives/carers and doctor to identify warning signs of relapse. Coping strategies and a crisis development plan can then be developed
4   The responsibility for prescribing and reviewing medication must be clearly defined between primary and secondary services. Anti-psychotic medication, particularly depots, should be reviewed at least every four to six months.

Table 13 Indications for prescribing

Drug Group	Indications
Oral anti-psychotics	Acute psychosis High levels of arousal Acute relapse of psychosis Continuing care: maintenance and prevention
Depot anti-psychotics	Continuing symptoms/difficulty remembering oral medication
Antimuscarinics	Only when side-effects (e.g. stiffness) are present
Lithium	Following third episode of manic-depressive illness, or to treat and prevent severe depression

(Adapted, with the author's permission, from Strathdee *et al.* *A General Practitioner's Guide to Managing Long-term Mental Health Disorders.* The Sainsbury Centre for Mental Health, 1996.)

Lithium monitoring

1 Lithium levels should be measured every three months; thyroid function and urea and electrolytes should also be checked
2 Levels should be taken 12 hours after the last dose. This is often most conveniently carried out at 10 a.m. after a 10 p.m. dose
3 Patients need to know the dangers of toxicity during an acute illness, when levels may build up quickly
4 Each patient should have a target range of allowable levels, based on experience of past effectiveness and side-effects.

Prescribing antidepressants

There is now a consensus about how depression should be treated in primary care, with guidelines from the Royal College of General Practitioners and Psychiatrists (Paykel & Priest, *British Medical Journal*, 1992). The main recommendation is to prescribe antidepressant medicine at effective doses for effective periods of time, thus improving patient outcome.

- at doses of 125–150 mg daily, tricyclic antidepressants are effective in patients in general practice with depressive illness
- there is *no* evidence from controlled trials that doses of 75 mg daily or lower are effective
- antidepressants have not been shown to be effective in the mild end of the clinical range of depression
- antidepressant medication can be used for moderate and severe depressions where, irrespective of cause, there is a persistent picture of the depressive syndrome
- four to six months of 'continuing' antidepressant therapy after the initial treatment phase helps prevent relapse
- for those with recurrent depression a 'prophylactic' dose of antidepressant as low as 75 mg tricyclic has been shown to be useful in preventing a further relapse. Lithium can also be considered in this situation

In spite of these guidelines GPs often prescribe low doses for short periods of time; this may be acceptable, if in the light of no improvement, doses are stepped up or treatments changed. Patients should ideally be informed about effectiveness and side-effects in order to be fully involved in decision making.

Appendix 3

The Care Programme Approach demystified

What is the Care Programme Approach (CPA)?

Developed by the Department of Health and introduced in 1991, the CPA aims to:

- prevent people with severe mental health problems 'falling through the net'
- offer a more systematic assessment of patients' needs with the identification of unmet need
- co-ordinate and integrate care from health, social services, housing and other agencies
- offer improvement in the quality of discharge planning
- promote shared care for mental health, enhancing inter-agency and multidisciplinary working
- facilitate care management and evidence-based clinical practice.

Those the CPA applies to

The CPA applies to those coming into contact with mental health services, usually prioritising those with severe mental health problems having complex needs. It is divided into three tiers:

Level 1 CPA (minimal). Level 1 is for people needing input from only one mental health professional. These cases may often be managed in primary care

Level 2 CPA (complex). Level 2 is for those needing input from two or more mental health professionals. In certain situations care may be based in general practice, given appropriate support.

Level 3 CPA (full, multidisciplinary). People on level 3 require input from a range of professionals and are at high risk or have very complex needs.

How does the CPA work?

Patients diagnosed with severe mental health problems by the responsible psychiatrist or social worker are placed on a local CPA list. Being on the list means that the patient will have:

- a key worker or named care co-ordinator
- an assessment of health and social needs
- an explicit care plan detailing the care providers
- regular care review meetings.

The CPA works effectively by:

- being integrated into routine clinical practice
- providing regular feedback to clinicians.

Care is planned in partnership with the people using the service and their carers.

What and who is a key worker or care co-ordinator?

A key worker or care co-ordinator may be any trained professional with mental health experience, including CPNs, occupational therapists, social workers, psychiatrists, psychologists and GPs. The key worker or care co-ordinator is responsible for:

- arranging needs assessments
- developing a care plan detailing the patient's needs
- monitoring this care plan and the patient's needs
- co-ordinating mental, physical and social care
- organising regular review meetings.

In some trusts key workers are support workers for those requiring extensive input and are not fully qualified mental health professionals. The term 'care co-ordinator' may be applied to those fulfilling the above statutory CPA functions.

Table 14 Key worker/care co-ordinator requirements and responsibilities

Level	Key worker requirements	Key worker responsibilities
Level 1	Anyone can act as key worker with agreement from the patient and multidisciplinary team (if appropriate), e.g. GP	1 To monitor and update the care plan as necessary 2 To keep other agencies informed of progress
Level 2	Any statutory organisation member who is part of the multidisciplinary team, e.g. social worker, CPN, etc.	1 Keep in close contact with the patient 2 Monitor that the agreed programme of care is delivered 3 To take immediate action if it is not 4 To invite all those involved in the patient's care to review meetings
Level 3	An experienced community health professional, e.g. approved social worker, psychologist	1 Ensure that the care plan adequately addresses the assessed risk/needs of the patient 2 The patient is assessed by the forensic team 3 The patient is given at least one-fifteenth of the key worker's clinical time

The benefits of multidisciplinary care (levels 2 and 3)

- everyone will have one named care co-ordinator and a contact telephone number
- the roles and responsibilities of each agency are clarified
- any shortfall in services can be identified and addressed
- appropriate services are made available to patients and their usefulness is regularly reviewed
- as a person's needs change, the service delivered to meet those needs must also change

Integrating primary health care teams into the CPA

- develop a joint list of people with severe mental health problems in each practice
- define roles and responsibilities of primary and secondary services
- agree a mutually accessible time and venue for CPA reviews
- develop agreed standardised CPA forms for written input
- develop CPA implementation training programmes
- organise CPAs in practices
- key workers/care co-ordinator should contact GP before CPAs

Appendix 4

Needs assessment and audit with paper records

The following form (Table 15) allows data to be collected for a needs assessment or audit of care. Suggested procedure for use is as follows:

- choose the items you wish to audit or measure need for from Table 15
- consider developing or using a long-term mental illness chronic disease card to collate the most important information for each patient; this can be kept in the notes as a clinical reference and for ongoing input. Alternatively, use a computer database
- use the Table 15 form to collate information on a sample of (for audit, at least 30), or all, patients
- for each patient whose notes are looked at
  - collate information on a chronic disease card or computer template
  - make any management decisions for that patient (e.g. letter to invite them for a mental health review)
  - place a mark on 'denominator' row
  - each time criteria are found, place a mark on the appropriate row (see the example of the 12 patients with bipolar affective disorder)
- calculate percentages by using Total number of notes audited as a denominator, e.g. 12/60 = 20 per cent of patients with LTMI have bipolar affective disorder
- finally, present and discuss findings as a team, in order to decide changes in care.

Table 15 Data sheet for needs assessment and audit of paper records

Criteria or need	Place a mark each time criteria or need is observed in notes	Total
e.g. bipolar affective disorder	⊺⊺⊺⊺ ⊺⊺⊺⊺ ‖	12

Total number of notes
    audited (= denominator):

Socio-demographic data
Male
Female
Ethnicity:
- Asian
- Black
- White
- Other

Home situation:
- lives alone – with help
- lives alone – no help
- lives with partner
- lives with family
- no fixed abode
- single parent

Next of kin/address/
    telephone no.

Clinical data
Diagnosis:
- schizophrenia/
  schizo-affective
- bipolar affective disorder
- psychosis (not otherwise
  specified)
- severe recurrent
  depression
- psychotic depression
- severe neurosis (e.g.
  PTSD, obsessive
  compulsive disorder,
  phobia, anxiety disorder)

History of deliberate self-harm

History of harm to others

Substance misuse recorded

Psychotropic medication
   recorded:
   • depot
   • Clozapine

CPA level :
   • 1
   • 2
   • 3
   • not specified

Service contact names
CPN/other community mental
   health worker specified: *Y/N*

Care co-ordinator specified: *Y/N*

Sharing of care
(first partner responsible for
overall needs assessment, recall,
mental state monitoring, risk
assessment, organising CPAs,
medication review and non-
urgent changes to medication)

Main care:
   • CMHT
   • GP
   • GP–CPN
   • Psychiatrist–GP
   • CMHT–GP
   • not specified

Other responsibilities
Lithium bloods:
   • CMHT
   • GP
   • not recorded

Lithium level interpretation and medication change:
- CMHT
- GP
- not recorded

Repeat prescribing:
- CMHT
- GP
- not recorded

Depot administration and recall:
- CMHT
- GP
- not recorded

Data input required on ongoing basis
Has each been recorded in the last 15 months?
Current mental state: *Y/N*
Medication reviewed: *Y/N*
Lithium levels checked in last six months: *Y/N*
Physical review: *Y/N*
CPA records in notes

Miscellaneous for audit
BP measured in last five years
Last BP <160/95
Smear up to date: *Y/N*

Example of a shared care agreement

Shared care agreement for patients with long-term mental health problems

This document is the written product of the process of negotiation and planning regarding care for patients with long-term mental illness registered with a practice. It documents the mutual agreement about how care will be provided by each party and across the primary–secondary interface. It particularly focuses on the model of shared care, the responsibilities undertaken and the methods of communication to be used. It also details the proposed developments in service provision and training. It is not designed to be a static arrangement; rather it is anticipated that with changes in the NHS, the practice and the trust, it will be reviewed.

Contact details

The Primary Health Care Team
Dr Bloggs' Surgery
Cherry Orchard Road
London, SW11
Tel.:
Bypass number:
Fax:

Staff
Dr Bloggs and Dr Smith (partners)
W Jones – Practice manager

J Black – Practice Nurse

Links with:

Community Mental Health Centre
London, SE

Case Management and Outreach Team
Team leader
Practice link worker
Part-time psychiatrist

The following types of mental illness are included:

- schizophrenia
- bipolar affective disorder
- psychosis (diagnosis not otherwise specified)
- psychotic depression
- severe depression (non-psychotic) (Severe recurrent depression and severe single episode causing substantial disability over a period of one year or more. Severe cases are likely to have had considerable agitation, retardation or suicidal intent.)
- eating disorders
- severe neurotic disorders (e.g. obsessive compulsive disorder, post traumatic stress disorder)
- personality disorders.

Many aspects of the agreement relate to practice policy and the practice plans to include patients on their register who have *dementia* and *drug* and *alcohol* problems. In terms of shared care, a different team will deal with these patients.

Shared priorities

The following specific priorities were established early in discussion:

- finding ways of helping carers
- focusing on identifying patients missing out on physical or mental health care
- improving information available in the practice and sharing this with

the community team
- improving understanding of how each team functions and working together more
- having a register to identify roles and gaps in care and to assist with commissioning.

Shared care arrangements

Linked liaison worker. A community mental health worker from the CMHT is linked to the practice and has limited responsibilities; he or she will primarily act to give advice and as a communication channel for the practice.

Should the link worker begin to preferentially take on cases from the practice?

The CMHT has a duty worker system, so urgent and general contact will best be done through that system. Urgent referrals will normally be seen at the emergency clinic. Occasionally, for cases known to the team it may be appropriate for patients to be seen at the CMHT base. Currently there is no 'fast track' method for seeing the community mental health team housing or benefits advisor.

Social work, benefits and housing advice. Patients with mental health related needs for housing or benefits would normally be referred to and assessed by the social work team. Where patients are able to take responsibility themselves they may also be referred directly by the practice. The practice should consider setting up a meeting with the social work team to explore shared concerns.

The following relationships within the shared care arrangement will be dominant and strengthened:

- community mental health worker (CMHW)–GP
- psychiatrist–GP
- CMHW–practice nurse.

Definition of roles and responsibilities

The role of the psychiatrist will include:

- urgent and non-urgent advice by telephone
- availability by bleep via CMHT or secretary
- consideration at allocation meetings of requests for direct out-patient appointments.

The role of attached/linked community mental health worker will include:

- discussion of possible referrals (all new referrals need to go to central team leader)
- providing general advice on patients with long-term mental illness, including those not under the CMHT or within CMHT boundaries
- providing general advice on the CMHT function
- accepting appropriate new referrals following discussion with team leader, as long as case load balance is not unduly affected
- giving advice regarding maintenance of case register
- access to practice notes/computer (for cases already known to the trust only)
- attending focused meetings at practice (twice monthly)
- liaising with the GP (as the responsible medical officer) to share care for more stable patients
- providing training to the practice.

The role of primary care in the Care Programme Approach process will include:

- occasional GP attendance at CPA meetings if very involved
- GP written input
- care co-ordinator/key worker contacting GP prior to CPA for discussion if required
- some CPA meetings to be held in the practice with GP attendance by prior arrangement.

The PHCT will provide the following physical care

- health promotion and disease prevention – recall for annual health check with practice nurse where patient is felt to potentially benefit
- opportunistic health promotion
- proactive investigation and referral for physical symptoms where appropriate
- liaison with key worker/carer to ensure attendance where appropriate
- giving of advice on obtaining care from opticians, chiropodists, dentists, etc.
- sending of copies of significant referrals for physical problems to the CMHT if the patient agrees. Letters could include a request for a copy of the appointment to be sent to the CMHT.

For those patients *not* under the trust/CMHT the GP's role will include following appropriate training on:

- mental state monitoring
- repeat prescribing
- medication review
- non-urgent changes to medication
- Lithium monitoring and medication changes
- recall for annual/quarterly review
- screening for mental health related needs, e.g. risk assessment, family and carer needs assessment, housing and benefits.

Responsibility for core community mental health activities will be recorded on a computer template. They include:

- overall needs assessment/screening
- mental state monitoring
- medication review and non-urgent medication changes
- Lithium and Carbamazepine bloods and associated medication changes
- prescribing repeat medication
- depot administration.

Communication content

Information required by the CMHT in referral letters:

- social and family background of patient
- explicit reason for referral
- responsibilities that the GP is willing to take on
- urgency of case (in weeks)
- medication and therapies received
- telephone number of patient

Information required by the PHCT in assessment, follow up and discharge letters:

- level of risk of harm, i.e. suicide, self-neglect, violence
- knowledge of patient and relatives/carers of the patient's condition
- predicted course of condition and its effect on the patient's lifestyle
- key worker's name and contact number, and whether the patient is on the CPA register
- management plan, including review date, objectives and outcome, anticipated roles of CMHT and PHCT
- definition of roles, including prescribing and monitoring responsibilities
- mental state on discharge, expected early signs of relapse and action to take
- group home/hostel address and contact number where applicable

Communication required during time of hospitalisation:

- fax of admission details to PHCT
- practice to be involved in discharge planning where appropriate
- information to practice regarding staged discharges and leave
- details of discharge faxed on the day of discharge
- essential details, including roles, to be clear and at head of discharge summary

Review:

The service developments planned will be reviewed at three months and the agreement will be reviewed in one year.

Signed on behalf of the practice...

Signed on behalf of the mental health team.......................................

References

Audit Commission. *Finding a place: A review of mental health services for adults*. London: HMSO, 1994.

Brugha, TS, Wing, JK & Smith, BL. Physical health of the long-term mentally ill in the community. Is there unmet need? *British Journal of Psychiatry* 1989; 155: 777–81.

Department of Health. *Building Bridges – A guide to arrangements for inter-agency working for the care and protection of severely mentally ill people*. London: Department of Health, 1995.

Dowrick, C. Improving mental health through primary care. *British Journal of General Practice* 1992; 42: 382–86.

Essex, B, Doig, R & Renshaw, J. Pilot study of records of shared care for people with mental illnesses. *British Medical Journal* 1990; 300: 1442–46.

Falloon, IRH, Shanahan, W, Laporta, M, *et al.* Integrated family, general practice and mental health care in the management of schizophrenia. *Journal of the Royal Society of Medicine* 1990; 83: 225–28.

Goldberg, D & Jackson, G. Interface between primary care and specialist mental health care. *British Journal of General Practice* 1992; 42: 267–69.

Grol, R. Implementing guidelines in general practice care. *Quality in Health Care* 1992; 1: 184–211.

Grol, R. Beliefs and evidence in changing clinical practice. *British Medical Journal* 1997; 315: 418–21.

Hampson, JP, Roberts, RI, & Morgan, DA. Shared care: a review of the literature. *Family Practice* 1996; 13(3): 264–79.

Honey, P, Mumford, A. *Manual of learning styles*. Berkshire: Honey and Mumford, 1986.

Kaeser, AC & Cooper, B. The psychiatric patient, the general practitioner and the out-patient clinic; and operational study: a review. *Psychological Medicine* 1971; 1: 312–25.

Kendrick, T, Sibbald, B, Burns, T & Freeling, P. Role of general practitioners in the care of long-term mentally ill patients. *British Medical Journal* 1991; 302: 508–10.

Kendrick, T, Burns, T, Freeling, P & Sibbald, B. Provision of care to general practice patients with disabling long-term mental illness: a survey in 16 practices. *British Journal of General Practice* 1994; 44: 301–05.

Kendrick, T, Burns, T & Freeling, P. Randomised controlled trial of teaching practitioners to carry out structured assessments of their long-term mentally ill patients. *British Medical Journal* 1995; 311: 93–98.

King, M, & Nazareth, I. Community care of patients with schizophrenia: the role of the primary health care team. *British Journal of General Practice* 1996; 46: 231–37.

King, MB. Management of schizophrenia – the general practitioner's role. *British Journal of General Practice* 1992; 42: 310–11.

Kolb, D. *Experiential learning*. New Jersey: Prentice-Hall, 1984.

Nazareth, I, King, M, & Davies, S. Care of schizophrenia in general practice: the general practitioner and the patient. *British Journal of General Practice* 1995; 45: 343–47.

Nazareth, ID & King, MB. Controlled evaluation of management of Schizophrenia in one general practice: A pilot study. *Family Practice* 1992; 9(2): 171–72.

Patmore, C & Weaver, J. *A Survey of Community Mental Health Centres*. London: Good Practices in Mental Health, 1990.

Paykel, ES & Priest, RG. Recognition and management of depression in general practice: consensus statement. *British Medical Journal* 1992; 305: 1198–1202.

Primary Healthcare Toolbox: Resource Pack. Health Education Authority, 1994.

Pullen, I & Yellowlees, AJ. Is communication improving between general practitioners and psychiatrists? *British Medical Journal* 1985; 290: 31–33.

Rogers, C. *Freedom to Learn.* Ohio: Merril, 1969.

Royal College of General Practitioners. *Shared care of patients with mental health problems. Report of a Joint Royal College Working Group.* Occasional Paper 60. London, 1993: 1–10.

Royal Colleges of Psychiatrists and General Practitioners. *Shared care of patients with mental health problems: A report of the Joint Royal College working group.* London: Royal Colleges of Psychiatrists and General Practitioners, 1993.

Strathdee, G. The GP, the community and shared psychiatric care. *The Practitioner* 1994; 238: 751–54.

Strathdee, G. Configuring Mental Health Services: A Needs Assessment Approach. In Thompson, K, Strathdee, G & Wood, H, eds. *Mental Health Service Development Skills Workbook.* London: The Sainsbury Centre for Mental Health, 1997.

Strathdee *et al.* *A General Practitioner's Guide to Managing Long-term Mental Health Disorders.* London: The Sainsbury Centre for Mental Health, 1996.

Sutherby, K & Szmukler, G. Crisis cards and self-help crisis initiative. *Psychiatric Bulletin* 1997; 22:4–7.

Thornicroft, G & Strathdee, G. *Commissioning Mental Health Services.* London: HMSO, 1996.

Williams, P & Wallace, BB. General practitioners and psychiatrists – do they communicate? *British Medical Journal* 1974; 1: 505.

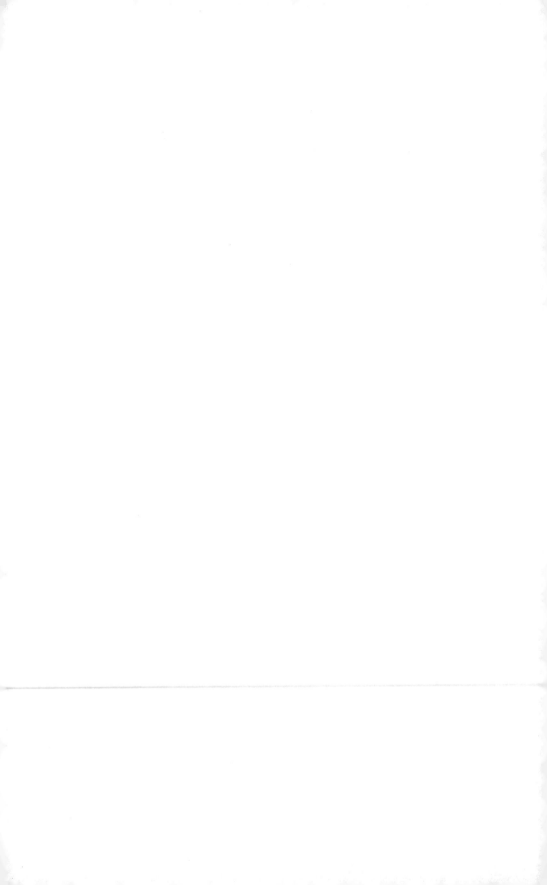